Stroke Rehabilitation

Stroke Rehabilitation

Structure and Strategy

Polly Laidler MCSP

Consultant editor: Jo Campling

CHAPMAN & HALL

London · Glasgow · Weinheim · New York · Tokyo · Melbourne · Madras

Published by Chapman & Hall, 2–6 Boundary Row, London, SE1 8HN, UK

Chapman & Hall, 2–6 Boundary Row, London SE1 8HN, UK

Blackie Academic & Professional, Wester Cleddens Road, Bishopbriggs, Glasgow G64 2NZ, UK

Chapman & Hall USA, One Penn Plaza, 41st Floor, New York NY 10119, USA

Chapman & Hall Japan, ITP Japan, Kyowa Building, 3F, 2-2-1 Hirakawacho, Chiyoda-ku, Tokyo 102, Japan

Chapman & Hall Australia, Thomas Nelson Australia, 102 Dodds Street, South Melbourne, Victoria 3205, Australia

Chapman & Hall India, R. Seshadri, 32 Second Main Road, CIT East, Madras 600 035, India

First edition 1994

©1994 Polly Laidler

This edition not for sale in North America and Australia; orders from these regions should be referred to Singular Publishing Group Inc., 4284 41st Street, San Diego, CA92105, USA

Typeset in 10/12 pt Palatino by EXPO Holdings, Malaysia
Printed in Great Britain by The Alden Press, Oxford

ISBN 0 412 46950 2

A catalogue record for this book is available from the British Library

Library of Congress Catalog Card Number: 94-70257

Contents

Preface

I have watched with growing concern the slow progress in matching new knowledge to clinical practice. In fact, as more research is undertaken and the frame of reference opens out to encompass the wealth of related, but hitherto neglected, issues, the gulfs are widening between academic 'researcher', 'specialist', 'practitioner' and the patient. As a member of the British Stroke Research Group, the British Society of Gerontology and relevant special interest groups of my own profession, and as a clinical practitioner specializing in, and teaching, stroke rehabilitation, the need to bridge these gaps becomes increasingly urgent. This book endeavours to provide some of the missing links in a logical format designed for all medical and related healthcare professionals, and yet which does not exclude other interested readers. **Don't skip the Introduction**, it answers some of the obvious questions and explains the layout and language.

My thanks go to all the stroke-survivors, and their families and friends, who taught me to question myself and my treatments, and to the many sources of expertise with whom I work or to whom I looked for their enlightened and specialized experience. I am particularly grateful to Dr Wayne Wilson PhD MA DipCST, Marie Napier (Social Worker), Helen Ellis DipCOT, Simon Wills BPharm MSc ACPP MRPharmS, Brenda Coward SRN (Continence Advisor), Kath Berney RGN DPSN, Dr Pam Enderby PhD MSc FCST, Dr Chris Gilleard PhD, Dr Geoffrey Kidd MSc PhD, Dr Peter Wilson MA BM BCh FRCP, Mr John Sutcliffe FRCS, Dr Alan Colchester PhD MRCP and Jenny Pennick; Gordon Maggs BSc, Jenny Strudwick BSc MCSP, Jackie Garratt DipCOT, Bill and Barbara Duke (stroke-survivor and partner) and Kate Hilliar BSc MCSP DipTP for their valuable advice and constructive criticism; Peter Razzell, Jean de Lemos, Geoffry Whitehead, Susan Brazzill and Tom Wright for the artwork and photography; and to John Hegley, whose poem gently sets the seal of infinite conjecture to the whole subject.

I am indebted to the publishers and authors who gave me permission to quote from or paraphase many excellent books and papers. These are duly attributed in the text and referenced at the close of each chapter. My thanks go also to Jo Campling, who persuaded me to write this book, and to Catherine Walker and Lisa Fraley of Chapman & Hall, who guided me gently through to publication. And finally, and especially, to Des, who has shared with me the course and conference absences and the frustrations and exultations, sadness and laughter resulting from my Need-To-Know the What, Why and How of stroke.

Polly Laidler
Wickham Bishops
1994

The Difference Between Truth and Adequacy

by John Hegley

Our Nature of Scientific Activity teacher
explained
that with scientific theories
NEAR is
sometimes close enough.
He gave the example of a law
of which science had been sure,
which had been obeyed
unquestioningly since it was made
but which was later discovered to ignore
certain variables;
sometimes what is seen as objective fact
is in fact only a rough guide,
which does the job of ordering
rather than DESCRIBING reality.
Applying this idea
to what is printed here
adequacy might say
'it's there in black and white',
whereas I think the truth would rather
cite
two shades of grey
of which one's extremely light.

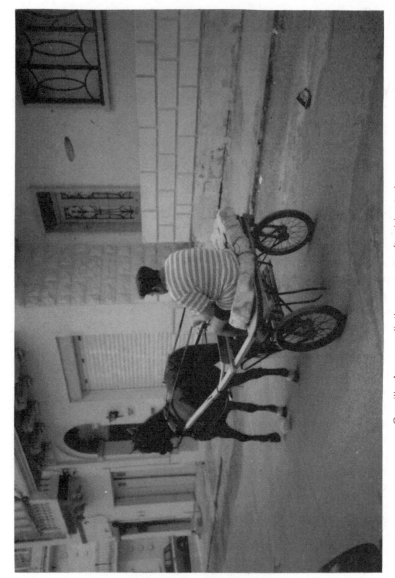

Camillo Azzopardi, three years after his stroke.

PART ONE
'What'

Introduction

The last decade has produced dramatic advances in the knowledge and understanding of the central nervous system, and the implications of these are wide-ranging and far-reaching. There are also pressures from changing economic, demographic, political and social systems forcing change in both administrative and clinical policies which affect the concept and provision of care. Economically and logistically, medical and caring services are overstretched and undermanned as a result. It is even more necessary, therefore, to review all the roles implicit in the management and care of patients and to apply a more pragmatic approach to these matters, bringing in more up-to-date knowledge in order to give a more satisfactory service.

The Need-To-Know much more of the What, Why and How of stroke is challenging the traditional modalities for all of us in the health care professions. Belatedly we are coming to realize that our professional training, in whichever discipline, is merely a baseline for 'continuing education'. From graduation, the applicability of our newly-acquired knowledge is being eroded (Zelikoff 1969). Dubin (1972) discusses the 'half-life of professional knowledge' and refers to an unpublished internal report by Rosenow (Vice President of the American College of Physicians) indicating that the half-life of medical knowledge is just 5 years: that after 10 years medical knowledge is only 25% as effective as at graduation. There is, therefore, an urgent need for education programmes to develop 'active learners for life' to facilitate life-long learning (Grant, 1992). Postgraduate education at present, whether formally or informally acquired, is more concerned with input than with evaluating the effect on output. At the World Congress of Physical Therapists in 1991, Ruth Grant warned: 'The hounds of obsolescence are nipping at our heels'.

Most of the definitive information currently available is too widely disseminated to be readily accessed by anyone who is already hard-pressed and over-committed in clinical practice. The following chapters incorporate an overview of many of the research findings, theories,

concepts and current thinking relevant to stroke, recovery and rehabilitation. One of the hitherto somewhat neglected areas that will be highlighted is the integral part that the nursing profession, domestic partners
and all carers play in the rehabilitation process. The management of
hospitalized or institutionalized stroke-survivors, and the handling and
expectations of those caring for the stroke-survivor at home, has a
profound influence on the degree of handicap resulting from the stroke.
In fact nurses and close carers are the primary rehabilitationists for
reasons which will become clear in Chapter 3.

The treatment of hemiplegic children cannot be included in a book on
adult hemiplegia. In children the early 'laying-down' of normal motor
behaviour is still to be – or is in the process of being – developed,
therefore any intervention requires specialist paediatric developmental
skills. However, once achieved, these patterns of motor behaviour
conform to identifiable norms and the disruption of these already-
established networks (as a result of specific or localized central nervous
system trauma) is interpreted in this book, together with the strategies
that may be appropriate to rehabilitation.

Action is meaningless without the substratum of the idea

Nick Miller, 1986.

Any textbook dealing merely with techniques is likely to be out-of-
date by the time it is published and in use. Therefore the purpose of this
book is not to prescribe but to describe, to update on the neurological
factors underlying the complexity of stroke, and to introduce the 'substratum of the idea', to enable both professionals and non-professionals
to evolve and progress their own special skills in assessment and
problem-solving to ensure ongoing recovery.

The content of each chapter contributes a platform upon which the
following chapter is based, to form an analogue of information on which
to build the personalized rehabilitation programmes required for each
individual Stroke. The references for each chapter are listed at the end of
each chapter, and a list of recommended further reading is given at the
end of the book. Medical terms – and some less familiar words – are
defined in the text and/or in the glossary. The book itself is in four parts:

- Part One 'What' explores the structuring, storage and retrieval of
  normal abilities in order to give a baseline from which to assess
  change following a stroke.
- Part Two 'Why' identifies and analyses these changes and surveys
  documentation and audit.
- Part Three 'How' describes rehabilitation strategies which overcome
  the major problems of stroke disablement, and discusses medical
  intervention and overall responsibility.

- Part Four 'Need-To-Know' includes selected (detailed) protocols vital to the management of early or severe strokes, lists of guidelines, a simple memo for non-medically-trained carers, and diagrams for quick reference and for use with relatives and other carers or for group teaching sessions (these are *aides-mémoire* only; the preceding chapters contain the knowledge with which to expand them appropriately), the glossary of terms used in the text, recommended reading, collected quotations and the index.

Much of the terminology used by medical personnel can be perplexing. 'Right-sided Stroke' for instance is used to describe not only the source of the problem (the right side of the brain) which actually refers to the left-side of the body being affected, but can also describe the right-side of the body affected by left-hemisphere damage. This, not surprisingly, confuses even the experts. Ongoing controversy over the most appropriate form of titling for anyone who does not conform to the medical standard of physical 'normality' makes writing a textbook on stroke even more of a hazardous undertaking! Personally I find the term 'patient' both patronizing and inaccurate, implying as it does that the individual needs to be receiving attention from others rather than reciprocating in a programme as an equal. To refer to the 'physically challenged' or 'less able' detracts from the specific nature of the handi-caps; 'stroke-impaired' is logical but long-winded when used repeti-tiously. In the text, therefore, in order to simplify communication and also to avoid arbitrary gender labelling, the person who has had the stroke will be called the **Stroke**. This is seen as the shortened form of 'the stroke-survivor', and is used purely to facilitate reading.

The side of the body affected by the stroke will be referred to as the 'stroke' (S) side – right (R) or left (L) – and the unaffected side (if there is one) will be called the 'non-stroke' (N) side because S and N can be visually interpreted faster (and are less distracting to read) than 'affected side' and 'unaffected side'.

'Hemiplegia' describes the unilateral effect of a stroke. Many Strokes display symptoms on both sides of the body, but if the signs of stroke are obviously unilateral they are likely to think of themselves as having a 'good' side and a 'bad' side, and this is psychologically damaging. Better to be honest but positive from the start, and refer primarily to their right and left sides – or, if describing stroke generally, the 'stroke side' and the 'other' (or non-stroke) side – in direct conversation with the client and family. Don't balk at the phrase 'stroke-sufferer' either as this is how the majority of stroke-survivors feel about themselves and their misfortune.

The line drawings are deliberately anonymous and mostly illustrate a Stroke with a L hemiplegia for the purpose of continuity. To apply them to Strokes with a R hemiplegia will require the reader to use their imagination (the visuospatial sketch pad in Chapter 4).

'Stroke' is formally defined in Chapter 1, but, in familiar terms:

> *a **stroke** is the result of a vascular accident in the central nervous system. It is a neurological disturbance of function often seen as affecting one side of the body. The site and extent of the damage in the central nervous system determines the laterality, severity and complexity of the ensuing problems.*

To the individual concerned it means loss or change – sometimes forever – of their 'normal' way of life. Any reduction in competence or independence presents not only a personal grief and deprivation, but also grief and loss for the families and friends who care for the disabled person.

Rehabilitationists need to understand and share this grief while working to alleviate it, but creating an awe-inspiring solemnity around the rehabilitation process is not the solution. Job satisfaction is not the prerogative of those employed to care and rehabilitate, either. The stroke-impaired are on the job 24-hours a day, seven days a week for as long as it takes (or for ever) and this has to be recognized. Make it enjoyable, lighten the load.

There is **life** to be lived after a stroke. It is time to renew interest and optimism in an area of work hitherto regarded as frustrating and often unrewarding for everyone concerned. This book is for everyone working with stroke-sufferers, in any setting, and in particular for those who find themselves without specialist support.

> *The important thing is to add life to years, not years to life.*
>
> *(Lord Amulree)*

REFERENCES

Dubin, S.S. (1972) Obsolescence or lifelong education: A choice for the professional. *American Psychologist*, **27**, 486–98.

Grant, R. (1992) Obsolescence or lifelong education: Choices and challenges. *Physiotherapy*, **78**(3), 167–71.

Miller, N. (1986) *Dyspraxia and its Management*, Croom Helm, London.

Zelikoff, S.B. (1969) On the obsolescence and retraining of engineering personnel. *Training and Development Journal*, **23**(4), 3–15.

The cause for concern

1

Little strokes fell great oaks ...

Benjamin Franklin

Statistics are indicators, not always accurate, and obviously subject to change as situations and the objectives of the statisticians alter. Statistics relating to stroke are no exception: mortality tables are easier to come by than morbidity (the incidence or numbers of people incurring a stroke), although both are skewed by inconsistencies relating to misdiagnoses or lack of accurate reporting. Many deaths attributed to bronchopneumonia, heart attack or merely old age may have actually occurred following stroke. Many 'mild' strokes may never be recognized as such and therefore may never be reported. The cause of a fall may be a slight stroke with temporary loss of balance reactions, but the fractured hip is the reason for admission to hospital, under the orthopaedic label.

Nevertheless, stroke is a huge and global problem with demographic variations in which the incidence is linked with that of coronary heart disease and other pathologies of the vascular system.

Stroke is the term employed to describe the acute neurological and irreversible (but not irremediable) manifestations of cerebrovascular disease which result from interruptions to blood flow in the brain. The World Health Organization defines stroke as involving 'rapidly developed clinical signs of focal or global disturbance of cerebral function, lasting more than 24 hours or leading to death, with no apparent cause other than a vascular origin'. Hemiplegias originating from head injury or neoplasm are excluded from the formal classification of stroke.

Reversible ischaemic neurological deficit (RIND) is defined as an event which lasts longer than 24 hours but recovers within 7 days – a 'minor' stroke (this is misleading as seen in Chapters 6 and 10).

TIA is **transient ischaemic attack**, which may present with all or some of the signs of stroke, but where the neurological deficits recover within 24 hours: the temporary cause (usually a small embolus) is quickly dispersed or dislodged to pass out of the system. However, a TIA, like a RIND, is an indication of cardio- or cerebro-vascular disease already presenting embolic or thrombotic matter, and is usually a precursor of a fullblown stroke if no measures are introduced to prevent it (Chapter 11).

Brain tissue depends for its survival on a continuous flow of blood providing it with oxygen and glucose and other essential nutrients. The blood supply is obtained from four main vessels, the right and left carotid arteries at the side of the throat and the two vertebral arteries which run up through the bones in the neck. These two pairs of major blood vessels, linked by the anterior and posterior communicating arteries, converge on the lower surface of the brain to form the 'circle of Willis'. From this point, blood is transported through the brain via a network of branch arteries.

Should a blockage occur in one of these arteries without being made good by a compensatory flow of blood from other vessels, the area of the brain served by the occluded artery will be deprived of its vital nutrition, resulting in tissue death. Infarction accounts for nearly three-quarters of all strokes, and involves processes similar to those underlying many heart attacks.

Arteries in the brain can be blocked by:

- the local development of clots (thromboses);
- the formation of deposits (atheromatous plaques) on the artery walls which narrow the channel until it is completely closed;
- the lodging of emboli (travelling debris such as dislodged pieces of plaques);
- thromboses formed elsewhere in the circulatory system following a heart attack, or during or after surgery for instance, which are unable to pass through the narrowed tubes.

The remaining quarter of strokes is caused by the leakage of blood from one of the arteries feeding the brain: the residual flow may not be sufficient, and the pooling blood will also create pressure on surrounding tissues. These haemorrhagic strokes result from weaknesses in the structure of artery walls – often hereditary – creating aneurysms which burst under stress (such as high blood pressure).

Cardiovascular diseases (CVD) account for a major proportion of all deaths during adulthood in both developed and developing countries. In developed countries they are responsible for 48% of all deaths, by far the greatest single known cause.

Atherosclerosis (the 'furring up' of the lining of artery walls) is the pathological process underlying thrombotic and embolic strokes; these strokes are major components of CVD tables in many countries (WHO technical report series 792, 1990). Although the mortality figures are lower now in certain regions than during the 1980s, possibly due to health education and disease prevention measures and increasingly sophisticated intervention, the overall morbidity figures have not fallen to the same extent. In fact there is some indication that there is an increase in non-fatal cases.

The World Health Organization (WHO) initiated the Comprehensive CVD Community Control programme in 1974 following a project in Finland two years earlier, targeting three already-identified high risk factors – elevated serum cholesterol levels, smoking and elevated blood pressure. The results have shown conclusively that cardiovascular mortality can be decreased by a community approach to control and prevention.

Dietary habits are significantly implicated, and high dietary fat intake appears to be the primary risk factor of the three. For instance, the Japanese remain a nation of heavy cigarette-smokers yet their place at the top of the CVD mortality league has dropped dramatically since a health education initiative succeeded in reducing the amount of salt in the national diet. In Scotland the incidence of CVD has dropped in an area where education efforts were aimed at increasing the amount of fresh fruit and vegetables in the diet and reducing fried food intake (and

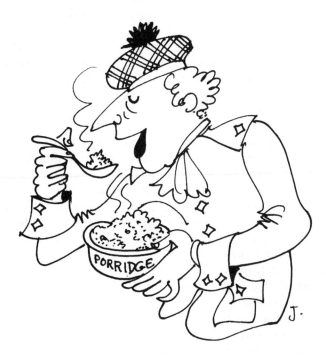

'Porridge is regaining popularity ...'

porridge is regaining popularity as the national dish because of its nutritional value!).

Increasing longevity is arousing international concern. In China by the year 2025 the average family is expected to be a couple with one child that has all four grandparents and three great-grandparents still living. In the USA life expectancy increased 140% between 1960 and 1980. Cerebral vascular disease affects approximately two percent of the civilian population in the United States. The rate of stroke incidence nearly doubles in every subsequent 10-year age group from 45 to 85. In England and Wales in 1991 there were an estimated 350,000 more people aged 75 and over than in 1985.

The incidence of stroke is heavily age-related – 50% of all strokes are in the over 75s – but although stroke is perceived to be a disease of the elderly, it can occur at any age and also *in utero*. It is the largest cause of serious disability in the developed countries of the world.

Figures for 1986 suggest that in England and Wales the toll of first strokes is around 102,000 persons per annum (equivalent to 2.4 per 1,000 population) and of these almost three out of five are female. In the UK there are estimated to be 150,000 disabled by it at any one time, 130,000 of these in private households. In 1988 the Office of Health Economics calculated that strokes cost the British National Health Service about £1 in every £25 spent – and this figure does not include the cost of home care or community support for survivors. A woman can spend 17 years caring for her children and another 18 years looking after aged dependants. If she has a stroke, the economic implications are distributed even further afield to include her care, the loss of her previous income, the care of her dependants and ongoing support; this saps both economic and manpower resources.

The prevalence of acute stroke in the United States has been estimated at 794 per 100,000 population, and costs American society over $7 billion per year in health care expenses, institutionalization and loss of manpower due to disability. Stroke survivors use up more days in short-stay hospitals than any other major diagnostic grouping.

In the United Kingdom it accounts for more than 60,000 deaths each year. Of those who survive, approximately one-third die within the first few days, one-third recover well enough to return home within 2 to 3 weeks, often without any medical or therapeutic intervention, and one-third remain severely disabled and need continuing care.

Hickey and Stilwell (1992) point out that 'the traditional indicators of morbidity and mortality provide only a limited description of the outcomes of chronic illness in older persons, and that identifying the numbers of people with specific chronic conditions fails to capture the wide variations in functional status and health service needs that exist among people with the same disease.' They go on to suggest that functional health is increasingly recognized as a more useful indicator than medical diagnosis of the health status of older adults, and that it is also a significant predictor of the use of health and social services.

For all these reasons it is now a matter of urgency that we find ways to delay or prevent the development, following a stroke, of unnecessary disability leading to dependency, to maximize recovery and to improve the quality of life.

In order to succeed it is necessary to expose a fundamental truth – that most of the chronic disabilities associated with stroke are acquired as a result of traditional management and doctrinaire techniques (i.e. a determination to apply a theory regardless of its practicability or consequences). Chapter 8 includes examples of these 'lame dogmas' and relates them to the data presented in Chapters 2, 3 and 4. The following sections present the other areas for concern:

1.1 Quality of life
1.2 Rehabilitation
1.3 Stroke rehabilitation
1.4 The psychology of adulthood

1.1 QUALITY OF LIFE

'Quality of life' was defined in a joint report by the Royal College of Nursing (UK) and the British Geriatric Society (1975) as:

> ... the ability of an individual to live to their own full potential as a human being.

In a further discussion, basic rights are described as 'recognition as an unique individual, with need for creative activity, the freedom to be alone or to enjoy the company of chosen others, and the right to be consulted – and to choose – in all matters affecting personal health, welfare and environment'.

It is valuable to explore this definition further in order to understand its relevence to rehabilitation in general, and to stroke in particular. As human beings we have certain primitive needs which must be met if we are to survive. Maslow (1954) postulated a hierarchy of needs in which 'higher' needs do not exist until lower needs are at least partially satisfied (Figure 1.1).

CREATIVITY

SELF-FULFILMENT

SOCIAL

SECURITY

PHYSIOLOGICAL

Figure 1.1 Maslow's hierarchy of needs.

This could explain some of the reactions, encountered during any rehabilitation process, that are commonly misdiagnosed as 'lack of motivation' (or just bloody-mindedness!). It must be difficult to get enthusiastic about being manhandled out of a 'secure' situation into a rickety wheelchair and bounced to the other side of the hospital in order to do a jigsaw puzzle (even if it is part of a formal perceptual retraining programme) with people you would not choose to be with, when you are more concerned about your unreliable bladder or being late for lunch.

In Maslow's understanding, security is lost and the physiological and social (both group and self-esteem) needs are seriously compromised, so self-fulfilment and creativity – and therefore motivation – in these circumstances are unattainable or, at best, considerably reduced.

The joint Report (Royal College of Nursing and British Geriatric Society, 1975) suggested that there are four basic requirements for quality of adult human life:

- Physical   functional health,
  mobility; preferably painfree and independent;
- Emotional   loving,
  being loved;
- Social   privacy,
  fellowship;
- Psychological   identity and freedom of choice.

Most people struck by stroke will be further desolated – particularly in hospital situations – by a sense of alienation from the rest of humankind. Their nearest and dearest may find it difficult to resume normal relationships with them. Mixed anxieties over health (the Stroke's), ability to cope (their own) and sometimes a genuine distaste for the altered physicality of a partner, can result in close family and friends withdrawing not only personal contact, but also the usual 'give and take' of family life and friendships so that emotional, social and psychological needs are impoverished in addition to any primary loss of normal functional movement and/or communication skills.

Rehabilitation is more than just dealing with the mobility and functional health of the disabled person; it has to encompass all the qualities of life and this necessitates reciprocal involvement with the individual concerned and with their family and friends. This is discussed further in Chapter 12.

1.2 REHABILITATION

Research into the effectiveness of stroke rehabilitation is gathering strength, but the whole field is riddled with pitfalls. Unlike the comparative simplicity of drug trials, electrotherapy or orthopaedic procedures, the rationale for remedial intervention in neurological conditions is wide open to interpretation. Is it the personal attention that raises the subject's level of motivation, the particular skills of that operator, or the specialized techniques being applied? The environment in which the studies are conducted? Could it be that the environment in which the subject is living, outside the trial, alters as a result of the inclusion factor itself (a known risk especially in randomized control trials)?

It is impossible to exclude these and other variables. Groups are almost impossible to match because of the infinite and individual variety of problems displayed by people with central nervous system trauma, and controlled studies are ethically vulnerable. Multiple single case studies offer rich pickings, but are considered unscientific and findings are usually rejected by the purists. Single case studies are now recognized as a useful source of information.

The term 'rehabilitation' has as many interpretations as there are rehabilitationists; the following definition includes most of them:

> an active process by which people disabled by injury or disease regain their former abilities or if full recovery is impossible, achieve their optimum physical, mental, social and vocational capacity and are integrated into the most appropriate environment of their choice.

There are, however, signs of an economically-induced dichotomy in rehabilitative goal-setting – a shift from the optimal restoration of ability to that of simplistic functional independence. At first sight this appears to be an alarmingly slippery slope and to present a disturbing ethical dilemma. The only goal-setting that rehabilitationists traditionally accept is that of achieving their patients' maximum potential for recovery – a subjective rather than an objective goal. Perhaps this apparent dichotomy can provide a new paradigm, a restructured concept of rehabilitation.

Hickey and Stilwell (1992) comment:

> 'The likelihood that prolonged chronic conditions will have negative effects on daily functioning emphasizes the importance of developing treatment strategies consistent with individual needs. The increasingly recognised importance of biosocial aspects of disease (especially in later life) suggests that health care providers may need to spend as much time addressing clients' beliefs and attitudes about illness and its consequences as they do providing clinical treatment for disease.'

A recent study by Partridge, Johnston and Morris (1991) found that elderly people's perceptions of their disability varied considerably from that of the professionals – general levels of activity and the ability to walk unaided were the factors most highly valued by the elderly group – and concluded that intervention should be explicitly related to individually perceived needs.

All this was admirably summed up at a joint conference held in the UK in 1991 by the College of Occupational Therapists and the Chartered Society of Physiotherapy:

> Possibly therapists should be directing their services to solving the problems which are important to their clients and not assuming that they understand or know what is best (Meredith, 1992).

With a new paradigm, the 'treatment' process could be defined as:

> any intervention, strategy, procedure or technique employed to help clients and their families, in partnership, to overcome, live with, manage, bypass, reduce or come to terms with the problems.

It is conceptually fluid, technically unbiased and indisputably pragmatic.

A client-led, rather than the conventional service-led, system would ensure that the two aims – the achievement of optimal potential and the restoration of basic functional independence – are not incompatible. Perhaps a more holistic statement, such as 'optimal restoration of functional health status' to replace the purely physical connotations, can reconcile the two objectives and achieve even better results. This is already the unstated philosophy underlying most home-based formal rehabilitation programmes, which are proving more successful than many hospital and outpatient-attendance schemes (Bryant *et al.*, 1974; Smyth, 1985).

1.3 STROKE REHABILITATION

Wade and Langton-Hewer (1983) suggest that admission into hospital is not necessarily essential for stroke victims, and family doctors (GPs) have indicated that the major factors underlying the need for hospital admission are the provision of nursing care, rehabilitation and adverse social conditions (Brocklehurst *et al.*, 1978; Bamford *et al.*, 1986). Certainly remaining in the home environment can be less traumatic for the Stroke, but there is a very real risk here that no referral will be made for rehabilitation – whether advisory or hands-on – until disablement is well advanced or even, in later stages, irreversible. With immediate intervention, however, activity can be clearly directed to 'optimal restoration of functional health status' in familiar surroundings and appropriate to individual need, and the family is included throughout which secures consistent and informed handling for optimum recovery (Chapter 10).

To enable someone to live with acquired disability requires a depth of teamwork and family involvement that is not catered for in the conventional medical model where clients are 'structured' into being patients, giving up their autonomy to 'the System', but seldom allowed to share it or given the help to regain it (Chapter 12).

Stroke rehabilitation is often characterized by the unpragmatic application of pre-determined fixed regimes and techniques, regardless of the result, to what is seen as an irreversible pathology – the inflexible in full pursuit of the unchangeable (with apologies to Oscar Wilde). But the problems of stroke are now known to be changeable (Chapter 3), therefore rehabilitation techniques must also be flexible and plastic. In other words, the recipients should not be moulded to fit into the current treatment trend as practised by their therapists, but the rehabilitation itself should be creatively tailored to each recipients' individual needs as these needs themselves evolve and change.

It has been said that once is a habit with physiotherapists! However you interpret it, this undoubtedly applies to anyone who is searching for the ultimate recipe for success: it is either discarded too soon or not soon enough.

There are other factors, too, that must be highlighted here:

- Failure to take into account the recipients' premorbid status. If he walked with a stick before his stroke, why expect him to walk without one afterwards? To satisfy a personal misconception of the Bobath Concept?
- Over-reaction to the premorbid status – if the client is crippled with rheumatoid arthritis prior to the stroke it does not mean that the stroke problems are insoluble.
- Failure to recognize the normal processes of ageing which run in parallel with acute and ongoing pathologies at any age. Behavioural problems may be only – or aggravated by – normal pubescent/ adolescent/senescent stages:

A manner rude and wild
Is common at your age …

Hilaire Belloc

Lethargy may be a genuine tiredness after eighty-something years of stressful existence – or a symptom of other pathological problems such as cardiac insufficiency.
- Failure to include the Stroke and the family and/or carers as active participants in the management and rehabilitation programmes.
- The assumption that any loss of independence through an acquired disability must also affect that person's adultness.

1.4 THE PSYCHOLOGY OF ADULTHOOD

Chris Gilleard (1992) suggests that adulthood involves three essential attributes, identity, autonomy and engagement:

- **identity** can be said to be: self or oneself, distinguishing character or personality, that by which to be recognized by others, self-recognition, individuality.
- **autonomy** is: independence, moral independence, self-determining, self-determined freedom, self-governing, paddling one's own canoe, self-direction, a degree of political independence possessed by a minority group.
- **engagement** in this context is: participation, to take part in, involvement, social interaction, to cause to mesh, meshed, and meshing.

Any one of these elements can be voluntarily relinquished and the dignity of adulthood retained.

Loss of autonomy alone is not significant; we are all accustomed to handing over our autonomy, both pre- and post-adulthood. In infancy it is in parental hands; in childhood it is shared between parent and school; in adolescence we are attempting to take control of our personal autonomy and learning to share it with others, at home, in school, college, university or career training schemes. As fully-fledged adults we voluntarily (however reluctantly!) relinquish our autonomy to managers or heads of departments, sometimes to partners, nearly always as a patient in hospital subjected to the in-house routines and hierarchies. When physically or mentally frail or disabled, much of this personal autonomy is of necessity given up to assorted carers, a Home or an institution. This does not create a problem if we can hold on to our personal identity and the ability to 'engage'.

Loss of identity leads to fragmentation and confusion, and the loss of engagement leads to disorientation and disengagement of social awareness.

This concept makes it easier to understand many of the apparent behavioural problems encountered in rehabilitation generally, and in stroke rehabilitation in particular. The adjustment from pre-stroke 'adulthood' with full autonomy, identity and free engagement, to a level of dependence that is seen collectively and individually as a global loss of adulthood itself, is a traumatic experience.

Of paramount importance is the need to recognize individual identity, and wherever possible to give a facility whereby this can be enhanced to make up for any reduced autonomy. Often physical handicaps are mistakenly perceived as a distortion of identity, or as an outward and visible sign of reduced adulthood. Maybe debating the Gilleard concept of adulthood could be appropriately therapeutic in these circumstances.

The freedom to engage and interact with others – also the freedom not to – is the other vital factor to take into account.

In a discussion of the concept as a baseline to a model of psychosocial dementia, Gilleard stated that the taking away of any of the three elements of adulthood is an infringement of human rights. Medical services are frequently guilty of doing so with physically disabled clients by their paternalistic (or maternalistic) approach to care. This certainly happens in care of the elderly: by depriving adults of their sense of adulthood, problems of orientation, confusion, dependency, depression and aggression become self-perpetuating and adversely affect progress. These are familiar obstacles when working with the stroke afflicted, too, and could well be induced by the care model itself.

TO SUMMARIZE

Think globally in every sense of the word. Quality of life, adulthood, attitudes and behaviours in and out of the rehabilitation context, are common denominators underlying all human relationships whether professional, personal, stroke-handicapped or not.

'There are strings,' said Mr Tappertit, '...in the human heart that had better not be wibrated.'

Charles Dickens (Barnaby Rudge)

REFERENCES

Bamford, J., Sandercock, P., Warlow, C. and Gray, M. (1986) Why are patients with acute stroke admitted to hospital? *British Medical Journal*, **292**, 1369–72.

Brocklehurst, J.C., Andrews, K., Morris, P., Richards, B.R. and Laycock, P.L. (1978) Why admit stroke patients to hospital? *Age and Ageing*, **7**, 100–107.

Bryant, N.H., Candland, L. and Loewenstein, R. (1974) Comparisons of care and cost outcomes for stroke patients with and without home care. *Stroke*, **5**, 54–9.

Royal College of Nursing and the British Geriatric Society (1975) Improving geriatric care in hospital. Guidelines.

Gilleard, C.J. (1992) Losing one's mind and losing one's place: a psychosocial model of dementia, in *Gerontology: responding to an ageing society*, (ed. K. Morgan), Jessica Kingsley, London, pp. 149–56.

Hickey, T. and Stilwell, D.L. (1992) Chronic illness and ageing: a personal-contextual model of age-related changes in health status. *Educational Gerontology*, **18**, 1–15.

Maslow, A.H. (1954) *Motivation and Personality*, Harper & Row, New York.

Meredith, B. (1992) report in *Physiotherapy*, **78**(2), 114–15.

Office of Health Economics (1988) Stroke. Report no. 89.

Partridge, C.J., Johnston, M. and Morris, L. (1991) Disability and Health Services: Perceptions, beliefs and experiences of elderly people, Centre for Physiotherapy Research, King's College, London.

OTHER SOURCE MATERIAL

Baum, H.M. (1982) Stroke prevalence: an analysis of data from the 1977 National Health Interview Survey. *Public Health Report*, **97**(24).

Effective Health Care (1992) 2: Stroke Rehabilitation. OIS University of Leeds, UK.

King's Fund Forum Consensus Statement (1988) The treatment of stroke. King's Fund Centre, London, UK.

The National Survey of Stroke (1981) USA.

National Center for Health Statistics (1979) Vital Health Statistics: utilisation of short stay hospitals. *U.S. Dept. Health, Educ., Welfare, Series 13 (41)*.

Smyth, L. (1985) Physiotherapy at home – does it help? *Physiotherapy*, **71**(9), 405–7.

Wade, D.T. and Langton-Hewer, R. (1983) Why admit stroke patients to hospital? *Lancet*, **1**, 807–9.

Construction of normal movement and ability

2

The nervous system regulates and integrates the systems of the body and it provides for the behaviour and intellectual attainments of man.
Murray Llewellyn Barr

Despite centuries of fascinated guesswork – and more formal scientific investigations into the working processes of non-human brains – remarkably little is known for certain about the human brain. Postmortem tissue gives static detail only, and experimental study of live human brains to find out what happens between the input and output is ethically limited! However, microtechnology and computer-generated picturing are becoming increasingly sophisticated and thus beginning to reveal more about the brain; what might be termed the 'morphological state of the art' is included here.

In conventional neurology, neuroanatomy and neurophysiology are dealt with as separate studies. The 'new' neurology is seen as a 'collective' field, and already many disciplines have merged under a common umbrella of 'biological sciences', 'biomedical sciences' or 'neurosciences' giving a biological base to psychology for the newly developing subjects of neuro-psychology and clinical neuro-psychology.

This chapter is a simple revision aiming to incorporate new material into a general framework to underpin the rest of the book. Only a brief outline is given of those areas particularly relevant to the understanding of stroke. The application of this knowledge to further awareness of all the processes involved in normal human activity is then detailed in appropriate subsections, which proceed, in a fairly natural sequence, from the following description of the nervous system itself.

The **nervous system** is a continuous tissue tract including all the neural structures, from the peripheral system (the nerves carrying information to and from individual muscles, joints, skin, etc.) to the **central nervous system** (CNS) which includes the **spinal cord** within the segmented vertebral column from which the peripheral nerves extend to their destinations, and the brain, protected within the bony cranium (Figure 2.1). This contains the **brainstem** (medulla, pons, cerebellum and mid-brain), the **diencephalon** (a complex collection of nuclei lying symmetrically on either side of the mid-line third ventricle in the depths of the cerebrum, including the thalamus and hypothalamus), and the **cerebrum** in the form of two cerebral hemispheres.

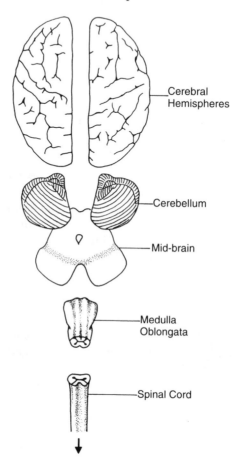

Figure 2.1 Basic structure of the CNS.

The **cerebral cortex** is the thin mantle (3–5 mm) of convoluted grey matter (approximately fifteen billion cell bodies) covering the surface of each cerebral hemisphere. It is believed to mediate all the human functions, including volitional control of many of the body activities, language, memory, geometric-, geographic- and self-perception, logical and illogical thought (Garoutte, 1987).

The **thalamus** serves as a relay station, a 'switchboard' for messages coming in from the sense organs. The massive thalamo-cortical interconnections are linked to speech and the control of sleep and wakefulness.

The **limbic system** is the term sometimes used to describe the structures around the central core of the brain closely interconnected with the hypothalamus; it appears to impose additional controls over some of the instinctive behaviours regulated by the hypothalamus and brainstem, and the emotional responses. The hippocampus is involved in the storage of new events in the memory for later recall.

The **cerebellum** coordinates, and is thought to be the library for, volitional motor functions. It is especially large in the human brain, receiving data from most of the sensory systems and the cerebral cortex, and eventually influencing motor neurons supplying the skeletal musculature. It influences muscle tonus in relation to posture, equilibrium, locomotion, and non-stereotyped movements based on individual experience (Barr and Kiernan, 1979).

Within the **brainstem** lie most of the auditory and vestibular (hearing and equilibratory) and oculomotor (eye movement) systems. 'These complex functions make possible the fine resolution and accuracy of the major senses' (Garoutte, 1987). The ventral portion of the pons provides for extensive connections between the cortex of a cerebral hemisphere and that of the contralateral (opposite) cerebellar hemisphere, for maximal efficiency of motor activity. The brainstem also mediates for the face the functions which are carried by the spinal cord for the rest of the body.

These higher centres of the CNS (Figure 2.2) generate, collect, collate, retrieve, discard and dispense all the information necessary for life to be lived.

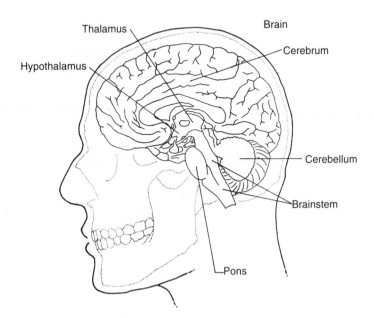

Figure 2.2 Higher centres of the CNS.

The **medulla** is continuous with the pons above and the spinal cord below. It carries all the ascending and descending tracts which communicate between the spinal cord and the brain. Just above the junction of the medulla with the spinal cord 80–90% of the corticospinal fibres decussate – those on the right crossing to the left, and vice versa – to form the lateral corticospinal tract in the lateral column of the spinal cord. Hence the reason that stroke damage in one half of the brain usually affects the other side of the body, and that brainstem strokes can affect both sides of the body.

The **spinal cord** relays sensory information from the peripheral nerves and motor 'action' impulses back to the same peripheral regions; some basic reflex mechanisms act directly through the spinal cord at segmental level, connecting sensory inputs with motor outputs without involving higher centres.

Spinal and **peripheral nervous tissue**, with its feeder blood vessels, is remarkably mobile. In the full 'slump' position (sitting with head slumped forwards on to the chest, trunk slumped as far forwards as the thighs

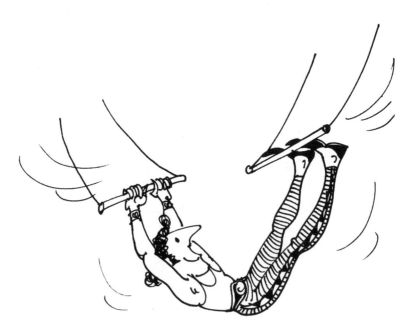

Spinal and peripheral nervous tissue has to be mobile.

allow and legs fully extended, feet and toes up) the mechanical stretch actually lengthens the spinal cord and peripheral nerves some five to eight centimetres (and can even exert a 'pull' on the brain stem structure), but after 15% elongation the walls of the feeder arteries are so narrow that adequate circulation is restricted (Chapters 6 and 10 relate posture to functional impairment). This freedom to move is both intra-neural (between the conducting fibres and their protective sheaths) and extra-neural (between the sheathed nerves and their immediate surroundings).

The whole system works by the transmission of impulses between cell bodies through their tendrils; this conducting unit is the **neuron** (Figure 2.3), and the masses of neuronal cell bodies form the grey matter of the brain and spinal cord. Dendrites are the cell processes for the reception of incoming nerve impulses to the neuronal cell body. The axon is the nerve fibre carrying impulses away from the neuronal cell body; in bulk the axons form the 'white matter' of the CNS. Typically, dendrites branch close to the cell body and axons remain singular for most of their course, only branching once well away from the parent cell.

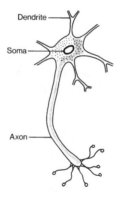

Figure 2.3 A neuron.

Synapses (Figure 2.4) are the sites of functional apposition between the conducting fibres of neurons – dendrite to dendrite, dendrite to axon, axon to axon or cell, and axons to effector organs (for example the neuro–muscular junction or 'endplate') – across which the messages are transmitted by complex processes of chemical and electrical polarization and de-polarization. Monosynaptic pathways conduct more rapidly than polysynaptic routes.

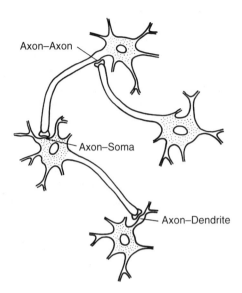

Figure 2.4 Synapses.

Presynaptic inhibition is the mechanism by which activity in spinal pathways is intercepted and controlled so that the ongoing message to the periphery incorporates all the feedback necessary for the resultant action to be both appropriate and accurate. Without presynaptic inhibition, muscle action is ungraded, resulting in a gross uncontrolled contraction (spasticity is described in Chapter 6).

Tracts are bundles of nerve fibres carrying information between the brain and the spinal cord; the medial reticulo-spinal tracts are considered to be concerned with the axial/proximal musculature of posture, and the lateral with voluntary distal actions.

Pathways are role-specific bundles of nerve fibres (afferent in/up, efferent out/down). In the CNS they are fed information from – or feed information into – the network of resource material at cortical and subcortical levels, etc. In the spinal cord they interconnect with local peripheral information systems. Excitation and inhibition (to further stimulate, or to damp down the stimulation to, action response) is coordinated again at this level.

In general terms the nervous system is clumped into two purposeful categories: somatic and autonomic.

Somatic systems are those pertaining to the body and controlling the striated (under volitional control) muscle tissue, in contrast to those associated with the viscera (the autonomic systems). Somatic neurons are classified by their roles: sensory, conveying afferent information from the peripheral sensory nerve endings up to the CNS, and motor, the efferent traffic from the CNS out to the periphery. Each basic pathway consists of three sensory, or a minimum of three motor, synapsing neurons.

The **autonomic system** is the part of the nervous system which controls the smooth muscle tissue for visceral functions of the body (respiration, digestion, circulation, excretion and the eye) and serve to maintain homeostasis (the body's physico-chemical equilibrium). It is almost completely autonomous and not usually subject to voluntary control. Two major subdivisions form the sympathetic and parasympathetic systems which are functionally related to their effects on homeostasis. For example, the **sympathetic system for** fight, fright, flight and the **parasympathetic system** for rest, recuperation and reproduction.

Little is known about the way in which the central nervous system exerts its control over the autonomic system; simple reflexes such as peristalsis (the travelling waves of constriction which propel food through the gut) are organized locally, others (vasodilation for example) at spinal level. General responses, such as those involved in the control of blood pressure, are integrated in the medulla and pons while adjustments to cope with situations (as in cardiac responses to exercise) are probably instigated by the frontal lobe and organized in the hypothalamus.

The **hypothalamus** governs eating, drinking and responses to stress-producing situations. It controls the endocrine systems and, in turn, the production of hormones. This concerns the mobilization of the complex physiological processes of 'fight-or-flight' reactions and the responses to intensely stressful physical exercise, for instance. The hypothalamus has been called the head ganglion of the autonomic nervous system (ganglion in this context being a cluster of cell bodies).

The following sections relate CNS control to human function:

2.1 Continence
2.2 Chewing and swallowing
2.3 Speech – phonation, resonance and articulation
2.4 Motor behaviour
2.5 Reflex activity
2.6 Postural control

Civilisation advances by extending the number of operations which we can perform without thinking about them.

Alfred North Whitehead

2.1 CONTINENCE

Somatic and autonomic systems, with some reflex activities, are all involved in the controlled excretion of body waste.

In infancy the sacral reflex arc allows emptying when the containing structures are full. With maturation and habituation this reflex emptying acquires CNS inhibitory control and the voiding of urine or evacuation of faeces becomes a voluntarily controlled action.

URINE The liquid waste processed by the kidneys is piped through the ureters into the bladder (Figure 2.5). The detrusor muscle forms the smooth muscle of the fundus of the bladder and is mounted on a firm base (the trigone) which includes the ureteric and internal urethral orifices. During filling, the detrusor accommodates an increasing volume of urine until the limit of the distensibility of the bladder is reached. The sensory data conveying the urge to void is processed and the response is organized on the 'Hamlet principle' ('To go or not to go, that is the question ...'). If the time and place are appropriate, then the fundus (under autonomic sympathetic system control) contracts, the flat base-plate of the trigone (under parasympathetic control) transforms into an open funnel leading into the urethra, and the external sphincter (under somatic control via the pudendal nerve) is relaxed to allow emptying. If time and place are not appropriate, the external sphincter contracts and the detrusor muscles remain relaxed until voiding is convenient.

FAECES The solid matter collects in the rectum and normal continence is achieved by the action of the internal and external anal sphincters and the flap valve formed by the right-angled anorectal junction: it is maintained by the puborectalis muscle of the pelvic floor.

The ano-rectal structure is composed of two tube-like components, one within the other. The inner is the termination of the alimentary viscus (viscera innervated by the autonomic nervous system). The outer component is somatic musculature forming the external anal sphincters; it is mainly reflexive, but is also subject to conscious control.

The internal sphincter maintains closure of the anal canal in the resting state: as flatus or faeces enter the anal canal, the external sphincter contracts until the appropriate time and place signals relaxation. If necessary, intra-abdominal pressure is then raised to expel the contents.

NORMAL MICTURITION AND DEFECATION

This involves the ability to store and to void urine and faeces at will, in suitable places and at convenient times, and it incorporates a cycle of events.

The normal cycle varies with age and custom, and between individuals: some find it normal to empty their bladder two-hourly, and others need to only twice a day.

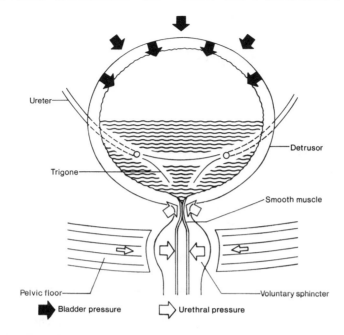

Ureter

Detrusor

Trigone

Smooth muscle

Pelvic floor

Voluntary sphincter

◆ Bladder pressure   ▷ Urethral pressure

Figure 2.5 The bladder, parts and pressures.
Reproduced with permission from Coloplast Ltd., Peterborough, UK.

The muscles of the pelvic floor have a dual role:

- unlike most skeletal muscle which generates activity only in response to stimulation, the pelvic floor musculature is constantly contracting, even during sleep, to combat the force of intra-abdominal pressure; the muscles additionally contract or relax according to circumstance. If intra-abdominal pressure rises as a result of coughing or lifting, for instance, which invokes a sudden strong abdominal muscle contraction, their tone is automatically reinforced to resist the pressure. Voluntary contraction can only be sustained for about 60 seconds.
- they play the most important part in the maintenance of continence by controlling the external sphincters.

Continence is defined as the ability to pass urine or faeces **voluntarily** in a socially acceptable place, and this depends on the successful completion of a sequence of five stages. A continent person is able to:

1. Recognize the need to 'go'
2. Identify the appropriate place to go
3. Get there

4. Hold on until it is appropriate to 'let go'
5. Let go.

Continence requires a complex interplay between autonomic, sensory and somatic nervous systems – and between spinal reflexes and higher CNS control. It depends on an intact and integrated neuromuscular system.

2.2 CHEWING AND SWALLOWING

The working components of the oro-pharynx are the lips, cheeks, tongue, soft palate, pharynx and larynx, involving all the complex networking of the somatic, sensory and autonomic systems. Sight, smell, touch, pressure, temperature, taste, proprioception, and learned responses, all affect the initiation of the voluntary and involuntary swallowing and respiratory mechanisms including the coordination of the muscles used in normal speech production.

The ability to eat and drink (**feeding**) starts, like all movement, with basic primitive reflex responses: the rooting and sucking reflexes which are triggered by brushing the side of the mouth or the cheek near the lips and subsequent pressure on the lips and tongue. This stimulates, in turn, an appropriate turning of the face towards the stimulation, opening of the mouth, closure of the lips on the entering of matter, and the use of the tongue to manipulate whatever is in the mouth. The soft palate is in the lowered position to keep everything in the front of the oral cavity at this stage (Figure 2.6(a)).

The swallow is initiated by the pressure of the food or fluid against the back of the throat, which stimulates the soft palate to elevate, creating a seal against the posterior pharyngeal wall which closes off the nasal cavities in anticipation of the swallow; then the tip and blade of the tongue come up to the hard palate, just behind the gums, to squeeze the contents backwards towards the pharynx, which in turn initiates the swallowing phase. The elevation of the soft palate is believed to stimulate the lifting of the larynx to create a firmer seal against the epiglottis to ensure that matter is not channelled down into the tracheal airway but passes safely into the oesophagus (Figure 2.6(b)).

The **gag reflex** is different to the swallow reflex: it is part of the protective mechanism and is stimulated by matter touching the fauces (the back of the oral cavity, between mouth and pharynx) too soon, before the swallow is initiated, to 'close' the throat. However the gag reflex does not always prevent matter entering the respiratory system; if it does, the **cough reflex** (a sharp expiratory 'explosion') is initiated to expel the substance from the airway. Note: air is held below the vocal cords under positive pressure when a swallow is initiated, in readiness for this 'explosive' release.

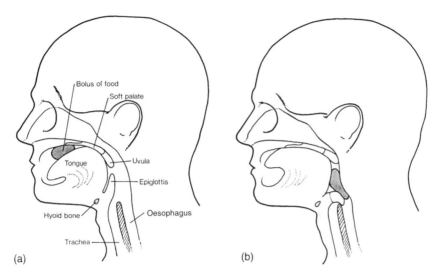

Figure 2.6 **(a)** Oral phase of swallowing: food bolus in the mouth;
(b) pharyngeal phase: bolus sliding over the epiglottis (which is sealing off the trachea) to pass safely into the oesophagus.

As maturation proceeds these reflexes are coordinated and modified into functional use, absorbing visual stimuli and acquired experience for control.

The **oral phase** is under voluntary control. The tongue, supported by pressure from the cheeks, operates to manipulate and direct the flow of food between the teeth or to spread liquid around the mouth. For mastication (chewing), the jaw moves up, down and sideways and saliva is produced to assist in the formation of a bolus (a lump suitable to swallow) by the tongue and cheeks. It is this bolus which is then further manipulated by the tongue to trigger the involuntary swallow.

The **pharyngeal phase** refers to the carriage of the bolus through the pharynx. The bolus is moved through the pharynx by the downward thrust of the tongue assisted by negative pressure in the pharynx and gravity.

The **oesophageal phase** describes the oesophageal peristalsis (muscular squeezing pattern) which transports the bolus through the cervical and thoracic sections of the oesophagus into the stomach.

A normal swallow, after the preparatory phase (i.e. chewing), takes five to ten seconds – less than a second each for the oral and pharyngeal phases, and three to seven seconds for the oesophageal phase. Most mouthfuls of food require several little swallows while liquid and saliva are extracted. The final swallowing is of the residual solid matter, the bolus itself.

Swallowing is not merely concerned with eating and drinking, of course: during waking hours any excess saliva is swallowed automatically, together with collections of post-nasal moisture.

2.3 SPEECH – PHONATION, RESONANCE AND ARTICULATION

[Language is cognitive and so covered in Chapter 4.]

Exhaled air is the power source for the production and realization of sounds, and for intonation, stressing, rhythm and phrasing. All the components of respiration from inspiration to exhalation, including the vital capacity (total volume of air) of the lungs, are essential to this purpose.

Phonation is the production of sound, involving the expelling of air from the lungs, through the vocal chords in the larynx (Figure 2.7) causing vibration which produces sound, and into the mouth which shapes the vibrating air to form meaningful sound.

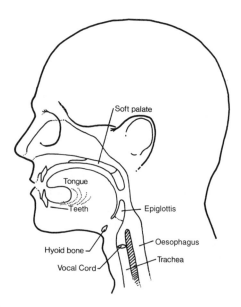

Figure 2.7 Structures involved in the production of speech.

Resonance gives quality to the sound; the mouth and hard palate acting as a variable baffle to reflect and project sound. Resonance varies with the movement of the soft palate in relation to the nasal cavities to increase or decrease nasality.

All the sounds for speech are made either with or without 'voice'. In a voiced sound the vocal chords vibrate together; in a voiceless sound air passes uninterrupted through the vocal folds and it is the articulators which form the desired sound.

Articulation is the way sound is manipulated by the tongue, teeth, lips and palate (the articulators) to produce identifiable and intelligible words.

Consonants are made – and made different from one another – by the way in which the teeth, tongue, lips and palate make and break contact with each other, and by their control and use of breath. For example, for 'b', 'p', 't', 'd', 'k' and the hard 'g', a plosive sound is necessary – produced by putting the lips firmly together, allowing air to build up behind the articulators and suddenly letting go, to allow the sound to explode forth.

The juxtaposition of the articulators enables differentiation. For instance:

- the lips mould   'p', 'b', 'm';
- lips and teeth   'f', 'v';
- tongue and teeth   'th', 'TH'.

The subtle variations in shape and position of the tongue against the hard palate create other consonants and sounds:

- tongue tip   'z', 't', 'd', 'l', 'n';
- mid-tongue   'ch', 'j', 'r', 'y', 'sh', 's', 'z';
- and back of tongue 'k', 'g'.

The difference between 'tar' and 'car', for instance, lies in the different placing of the tongue.

Vowels are made with uninterrupted voiced air by changing the shape of the mouth using the lips and tongue: the air flow is not stopped or constricted in any way.

The production of intelligible speech depends on sophisticated and complex processing, organization and coordination of the somatic, sensory and autonomic systems involving respiration, laryngeal and palatal structures, tongue, lips, jaw and cheeks.

2.4 MOTOR BEHAVIOUR

What we have to learn to do, we learn by doing.

Aristotle

We move in response to a need to move, either to a sensory trigger:

- tactile (skin sensation: touch, temperature, pain);
- proprioceptive (uncomfortable joint position, muscle or tendon stretch);
- visual (a static or moving object, person, light);
- auditory (sound);
- olfactory (smell, food, burning);

or to a cognitive 'executive' initiative (for instance memory/time-related: 'The meeting starts in half-an-hour so I've just got time for a shower').

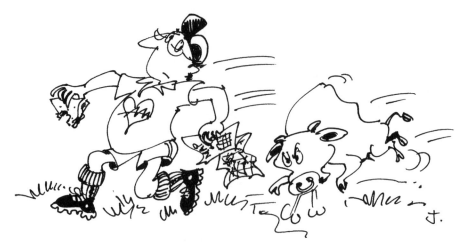

We move in response to a need to move ...

Sensory input to the spinal cord along the dorsal roots from cutaneous (skin), muscle, joint and deep fascial receptors not only provides information for the ascending sensory pathways, but may also elicit reflex responses employing collateral connections with interneurons and motor neurons in the grey matter of the spinal cord. The incoming data is received, processed and organized by the central nervous system and is then transmitted as complex volleys of 'action potential' to synapses with spinal cord alpha and gamma anterior horn cells, and with excitatory and inhibitory interneurons, to activate rhythmic contractions of the motor units of the primary agonist (mover) and synergist (supporter) muscles needed for the movement, together with simultaneous graded inhibition of the antagonists (opposing groups). This also adjusts the reflex reactivity of alpha anterior horn cells, the gamma system and Golgi tendon organs, to smooth the contractions.

The resulting voluntary movement can only proceed if anticipated by – or concomitant with – the appropriate postural adjustments necessary to maintain central stability against gravity.

We learn to move by experiencing movement, by trial and error until the required goal is achieved with maximum efficiency and minimum energy expenditure. This applies to all functional activity, from learning to hold the head up in babyhood to sophisticated skills like juggling plates while riding a unicycle.

The truth of the old sayings 'practice makes perfect' and 'use it or lose it' is now scientifically proven, in studies of the **Purkinje cell** in the cerebellum for instance. This cell responds to repeated similar impulses by sprouting a new dendrite: the more it receives the greater the growth, and vice versa. If the input ceases before full growth is complete, the new sprouts shrink back again. Volleys of different impulses stimulate other new dendrite sprouts.

New working synapses evolve in seven days, so the sequencing of the components making up successful movement is then 'on network' in the CNS and with sufficient repetition eventually forms an 'automatic' responsive background for inclusion into other movements.

The somatic afferent–efferent (input/output) conversion is no longer seen in terms of simple geographical locations of 'sensory cortex' and 'motor cortex' – for instance, only one-third of 'efferent' motor fibres actually originates in the 'motor cortex' – but as a complex hierarchy of dynamic cross-referencing systems (Figure 2.8), processing from the initiating trigger to the completion of the movement by trawling:

- memory and executive planning;
- continuing sensory and vestibular information (from the 'gyroscopic' mechanism in the internal ear);
- acquired 'sets' of learned movement and changing tonus (the inhibition and excitation of inhibition and excitation of muscle tissue);
- reciprocal innervation;
- reflex inhibition and excitation;
- and so on.

The processing from GO to GOAL is estimated to take 10–20 μs (millionths of a second).

Nigel Lawes, lecturing in 1991, stated cheerfully that the concept of the extrapyramidal system is no longer valid and that the function of the rubrospinal tract in humans is in doubt; that the corticospinal tracts are not just motor pathways, but modify both input and output, and motor/sensory areas can be activated to stimulate each other, as in eye movements, for example. The eye moves to see: if still unable to see, then a global body movement is generated to expand the field of vision, to enable seeing. 'Gaze control' is explored in section 2.6.

J.F. Stein (1982) defines two forms of movement control, 'open loop' and 'closed loop'. **Open loop 'ballistic' control** is completely pre-programmed and completed independently whatever may happen during execution. This enables a very fast response but it can be faulty, due to a lack of time to monitor internal or external changes, e.g. swatting a fly and missing it, because the fly flew off after the spontaneous 'automatic' movement response was activated. **Extended closed loop 'pursuit' control**, can be compared with other scientific engineering designs like heat-seeking missiles; it is servo-assisted motor behaviour! It is slower but accurate, utilizing continuous feedback from both internal and external sources, e.g. for walking on uneven ground.

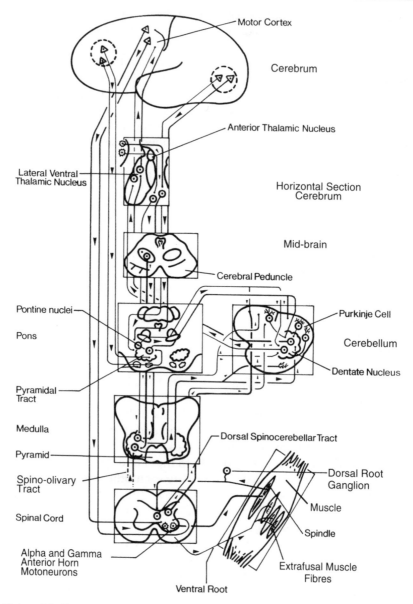

Figure 2.8 Some of the complex trafficking in the CNS (after Garoutte, 1987).

Most movement is initiated ballistically but finishes with corrective feedback control to attain the goal or objective. It also requires a predictive element based on previous experience, e.g. fly-swatting and getting it!

Normal adult movement is 'pre-packed', dependent upon integrated CNS control for all functional activity. This entirely neurological perspective is augmented by a cognitive processing system, such as the model described in Chapter 4, which illuminates the concept of normal movement and its disorders.

2.5 REFLEX ACTIVITY

Man is one chain of excitation surrounded by a wall of inhibition.
                                                    Charles Scott Sherrington

A primitive reflex is an involuntary motor response, at spinal-segmental level, to a sensory stimulus. For example, the knee-jerk reaction to a sharp tap below the patella is an instant muscle contraction in response to the momentary tendon-stretch; it is an unmonitored basic monophasic reflex arc 'hard-wired' into the spinal cord.

More complex are the stereotyped responses involving primitive patterns of movement.

The **stereotyped reflexes** particularly associated with stroke are those of flexion or extension of the entire limb, with rotation at those joints which allow it. Stein (1982) described 'open-loop' reflexes – in which the stimulus triggers a sequence of actions not regulated by feedback, e.g. the flexion 'withdrawal' reflex – and 'closed-loop' reflexes – where the stimulus regulates the degree of muscle contraction and is itself affected by the response, which in turn refeeds back on the stimulus, e.g. control of the stretch reflex mechanism in muscle tissue, involving interaction between local excitation and inhibition, and between spinal reflex activity and higher control.

Automatic movements are the programmed responses acquired through the consistent use of specific actions which form neuronal sets (or 'pools') at spinal level through several segments. These produce a coordinated pattern of muscle actions initiated at the periphery and regulated by local and higher centres.

Earlier animal studies have shown that basic movement patterns such as quadrupedal gait, generated by the spinal cord programmes of movement, are initiated and modified by input from both the CNS and from the periphery (Grillner, 1981, provides a review). This modifying input from the periphery appears to come from proximal regions of the limbs, but the receptors responsible have not been identified; they may be associated with joint, skin or muscle (Anderson *et al.*, 1978; Rossignol and Gauthier, 1980). Lundberg (1979) suggests that the different afferents converging at an interneural spinal level form multisensory reflex feedback systems.

In humans, the descending inhibition of interneurons from the CNS by a presynaptic inhibitory mechanism could be augmented by this second peripheral segmental presynaptic inhibition. Bobath observed in 1978 that movement or change in position of proximal limb joints can reduce spasticity and facilitate movement. Musa (1986) proposes that if supra-segmental presynaptic inhibition is lost due to damage to higher centres, this segmental inhibitory mechanism can act on spinal reflex pathways – that this secondary segmental system of presynaptic inhibition may then be the only way of switching on presynaptic inhibitory mechanisms.

2.6 POSTURAL CONTROL

When you are down, everything falls on you.

(Sylvia Townsend Warner)

The factor around which all functional movement evolves is gravity. The weight of a body is the force exerted on it by the Earth's gravitational field; the common measure of the Earth's gravitational field is the rate at which a free-falling object accelerates – 9.8 metres per second per second (32 feet per second per second). This remains constant whatever the mass of the object.

Evolutionary transition from quadruped to biped not only freed the forelimbs from a supporting role to develop selective and sophisticated

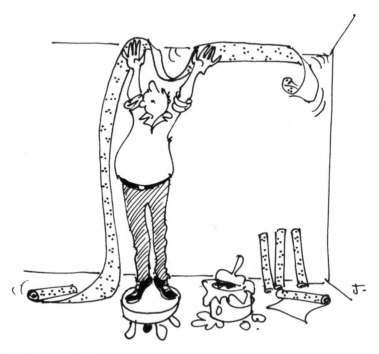

... freed the forelimbs to develop selective and sophisticated control ...

skills, but also necessitated a complete rethink of the control of musculature to cope with the gravitational forces acting on the newly destabilized body: a taller, infinitely more mobile, vertical model supported from underneath by just two legs (instead of the short horizontal creature stabilized by a leg at each corner).

The control of posture against gravity is developed from birth onwards – from the moment the infant is exposed to the Earth's gravitational field. The establishing of the normal postural mechanism is achieved through postnatal experience.

Berta Bobath (1990) placed the primary responses to gravity into three groups:

- **righting reactions** which serve to maintain and restore the position of the head in space (face vertical, mouth and eyes horizontal) and its normal relationship with the trunk together with the normal alignment of trunk and limbs. These reactions are well-advanced by the age of five months to include rotation round the body axis.
- **equilibrium reactions** which serve to maintain and restore balance during all activity by the use of counter-movements in relation to the degree of disturbance of the body's own centre of gravity. These reactions should be well coordinated by the age of seven years.
- **automatic adaptation** of muscles to change of posture; this involves reciprocal innervation and the grading of muscle tone (normal muscle tone is described as being high enough to withstand gravity, but low enough to allow movement).

The major anti-gravity muscle groups are those of the trunk (from head to hip) and the legs. Their role is to extend the body and hold the weight of the erect body column against gravity. Primarily these are the back and buttock muscles of the trunk and hips, and the quadriceps at the front of the thighs, perhaps philogenetically coded from primitive four-legged beginnings when head raising against gravity was paramout followed in evolution by the necessity to rear up on to the hind legs and stay upright on braced knees.

The abdominal muscles work in a slightly lesser capacity to hold the thorax to the front of the pelvis in order to support and maintain the erect position. Dr Karel Bobath, explaining the strong flexor reflex patterns, throws in the idea that our early forbears also needed to grab a branch of the nearest tree and pull themselves up out of reach of ravenous carnivores!

The anti-gravity muscles are the strongest muscle groups; their trophic code (genetic protein code) determines that their muscle fibres are red SO – predominantly slow-fatiguing and extra-rich in oxygenated blood – the relevance of this physiology will be explained in Chapter 3.

We are able to make postural adjustments without involving any specific peripheral limb movement, as in wriggling into a more comfortable sitting position, but the converse activity is impossible in the normally-developed adult – no effective voluntary movement distally is possible without corresponding postural adaptations to give central stability against gravity. Without postural adjustment even raising an arm would topple the body off-balance. These dynamic changes may not be obvious – they are predominantly due to subtle complex variations in muscle tonus.

Biomechanical factors are integral in the consideration of postural control. This extract describing the biomechanical implications is taken from a paper by Butler and Major (1992): 'The individual segments (sections) that comprise the head, trunk, and lower limbs (if standing) form a weight-bearing vertical column within the gravitational field. Movement is a primary objective of the human body and is achieved by means of this multi-segmented articulated structure. Most movements performed within a gravitational field require a reaction external to the body; this reaction is usually provided by the ground. The body obtains these external reactions through a pseudo-fixed base – for example the feet in walking – while maintaining dynamic control of the entire column of joints and segments above the base. By means of this dynamic control, each segment is maintained in an orientation which is appropriate to support all the segments that are above. Mechanical stability would easily be lost were it not for the neurophysiological control system incorporating rich feedback mechanisms. Each segment of the vertical column is influenced by forces from other segments both above and below the one in question; thus accurate controlled movements in the vertical posture can take place only if the correct control strategies are operating throughout the entire weight-bearing column of segments. These normal correct control strategies enable accurate (precise and efficient) movement to take place in situations of different control complexity; these situations range from maintenance of a static unperturbed posture of the segmental column to the most demanding control situation in which external perturbations are superimposed on voluntary movement, as in walking through a moving railway carriage'.

In biomechanical terms, the execution of an accurate movement incorporates three main aspects (Butler and Major, 1992):

- there must be accurate determination of the position of the body in the gravitational field, coupled with the control system having knowledge of the relative position of joints controlling the relationship of body segments.
- the movement must be planned, taking due account of the desired goal.
- the movement itself is carried out together with any postural adjustments required to maintain stability in the presence of dynamic reactions.

The concept of 'centre of mass' used in therapeutic analyses of function and movement of the human body is inappropriate when considering the mobility or stability of the complex multi-segmented human structure at a particular support point (Major and Butler, 1991). Their proposed alternative is **instantaneous supported mass effect** (ISME), which is obviously essential for accurate reporting and detailed analysis. However, for general purposes, this book will continue to refer to the somewhat old-fashioned notion of a **centre of gravity** (CoG), and place this 'centre of gravity' – for stroke rehabilitation purposes – somewhere in the mid-lower thoracic region of the average adult; this is the centre of body mass above the hip joints. Bobath tutors suggest it could be imagined as being between the tip of the sternum and the body of the 11th thoracic vertebra, and identify it as the central 'key point' in the rehabilitation of impaired movement control.

Displacement of this centre of gravity produces the coordinated counter-balancing responses of 'equilibrium reactions': when leaning backwards on a bar stool, for instance, the legs lift forwards (drunks, unable to respond fast enough, flail about or fall off).

In **neurological** terms, Carr and Shepherd (1989) summarize three major findings from recent research programmes which show that postural adjustments are:

- **anticipatory and ongoing,** e.g. preparatory adjustments ensure that the potentially destabilizing effect of an arm movement is countered before it occurs;
- **task- and context-specific,** i.e. muscle activation patterns vary according to the position of the individual, the task being performed and the context in which it occurs;
- **visually-affected,** i.e. vision provides critical information about body position in space, which is of course directly relevant to the anticipatory element.

GAZE CONTROL

During a discussion on posture control in cerebral palsy children in 1991, Alain Berthoz suggested that the way some of these children roll the head and eyes prior to extending neck and head into a relatively stable erect position could be related to the use of vision to stimulate other impaired motor pathways; that they are searching visually for a high fixed point distally and then by forcing their eyes upwards to this point are able to trigger the required motor action. By offering a visual marker, such as a bright toy, to obtain visual focus and then raising it slowly, the child is often able to lift the head more directly.

In normal adults the appropriate position of the head in space is primarily achieved by the processing of information from the vestibular systems to create a spatial 'centre' – an inertial guidance platform using the ground as the frame of reference – which stabilizes the retinar image for running on even ground, for instance. The angle of gaze is projected along the line drawn from the meatus of the ear to the midline of the eyesocket, and it centres the visual field. The angle of the head during activity varies and is determined by task (Figure 2.9); for instance it is gaze-dependent for intermittent stability during complex movements, e.g. gaze control directs skiing over uneven ground by ensuring that the legs 'lift' into flexion first in order to ride the lesser bumps instead of extending to exert 'push' to jump them.

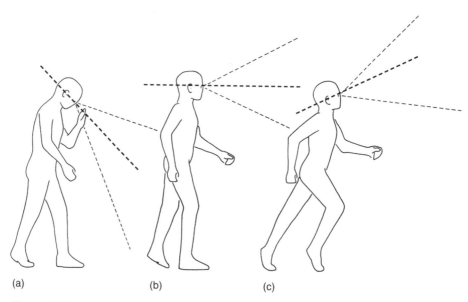

(a)   (b)   (c)

Figure 2.9 (a to c) Gaze-controlled head posture during movement.

Visual pathways take over when tactile and proprioceptive information is impaired: the direction of gaze angles down to assess immediate ground surface to facilitate locomotion. Other stabilizing means are utilized to enhance (and where necessary replace) the vestibulo-spinal and visual pathways: sensory information from heel-strike, for example. In the dark, length of stride shortens to increase the frequency and accuracy of other sensory input in order to determine ground surface stability.

We think in generalities, but we live in detail.

(Alfred North Whitehead)

REFERENCES

Anderson, O., Grillner, S., Lindquist, M. and Zomlefer, M. (1978) Peripheral control of the spinal pattern generators for locomotion in cats. *Brain Research*, **150**, 625–30.

Barr, M.L. and Kiernan, J.A. (1979) *The Human Nervous System*, 5th edn, Harper International, New York.

Bobath, B. (1990) *Adult Hemiplegia: evaluation and treatment*, 3rd edn, Heinemann, London.

Butler, P.B. and Major, R.E. (1992) The learning of motor control: biomechanical considerations. *Physiotherapy*, **78**(1), 6–10.

Carr, J.H. and Shepherd, R.B. (1989) A motor learning model for stroke rehabilitation. *Physiotherapy*, **75**(7), 372–80.

Garoutte, B. (1987) *Survey of Functional Neuroanatomy*, 2nd edn, Jones Medical Publications, Greenbrae CA.

Grillner, S. (1981) Control of locomotion in bipeds, tetrapods and fish, in *Handbook of Physiology Vol III, section I: the nervous system II, motor control* (ed. V. Brooks), American Physiological Society, Waverley Press, Baltimore, pp. 1179–236.

Lundberg, A. (1979) Multisensory control of spinal reflex pathways. *Progress in Brain research*, **50**, 11–28.

Major, R.E. and Butler, P.B. (1991) Instantaneous supported mass effect ISME: an alternative to centre of mass in discussion of the human structure. *Clinical Rehabilitation*, **5**(1), 87–8.

Musa, I.M. (1986) The role of afferent input in the reduction of spasticity: an hypothesis. *Physiotherapy*, **72**(4), 179–82.

Rossignol, S. and Gauthier, L. (1980) An analysis of mechanisms controlling the reversal of crossed spinal reflexes. *Brain Research*, **182**, 31–45.

Stein, J.F. (1982) *An Introduction to Neurophysiology*, Blackwell, Oxford.

OTHER SOURCE MATERIAL

Berthoz, A. and Pozzo, T. (1988) Intermittent head stabilisation during postural and locomotory tasks in humans, in *Posture and Gait: development, adaptation and modulation*, (eds B. Amblard, A. Berthoz and F. Clarac), Elsevier, Amsterdam, pp. 189–98.

Carr, J.H. and Shepherd, R.B. (1990) A motor learning model for rehabilitation of the movement-disabled, in *Key Issues in Neurological Physiotherapy*, (eds L. Ada and C. Canning), Butterworth–Heinnemann, Oxford, pp. 1–24.

Enderby, P. (1984) Assisting the patient who has difficulty with swallowing. *Bulletin of the College of Speech Therapists*, **388**, 1–3.

Pozzo, T., Berthoz, A. and Lefort, L. (1990) Head stabilisation during various locomotor tasks in humans: 1: normal subjects. *Experimental Brain Research*, **82**, 7–106.

Neuromuscular plasticity

3

... that to live is to change, and to be perfect is to have changed often.

(*Cardinal Newman*)

Plasticity is the ability of cells to alter any aspect of their **phenotype** (their 'gene expression' – the physical, biochemical and physiological coding determined genetically and environmentally), at any stage in their development, in response to abnormal changes (intracellular or extracellular) in their state or environment (Brown and Hardman, 1987).

Walshe stated that the brain knows nothing of muscles, only of movement: the brain is now understood to control the attainment of motor goals. Motor goals are cyclic. The actions required for the performance of a movement are not only modified and improved in time to reach the goal even as its 'goalposts' are moving (extended closed-loop 'ballistic' control), and the trace of the activity recorded for replay, but if the goal and/or the performance are found to be inadequate the performance and the goal can be extended further in time and space in order to achieve a successful outcome (e.g. a heat-seeking missile changing targets).

This chapter holds the key to all effective rehabilitation. The physiological detail may seem grossly simplistic to some readers (and somewhat daunting to others), but stay with it!

3.1 Function-induced plastic adaptability
3.2 Physiological stressing
3.3 Enable or disable
3.4 Electrical neuromuscular stimulation.

3.1 FUNCTION-INDUCED PLASTIC ADAPTABILITY

Skeletal muscle is striated, composed of many individual fibres each of which is a long multinucleated cell of varying length and width containing contractile myofibrils. Homogeneous muscle fibres are bundled together and each bundle is innervated by a motoneuron to form a motor unit. The contractile and metabolic properties of the motor units are determined by their respective motor nerves. (Buller *et al.*, 1960)

Cardiac muscle fibres contain only one, or sometimes two, nuclei and myofibrils, and are therefore somewhere between 'smooth' (having one nucleus) and 'striated'.

Proteins are the principal constituents of the protoplasm of all cells, and each protein has a unique genetically-defined amino acid sequence which determines its specific shape and function. The trophic code of muscle tissue is dynamic – the proteins are held in a dynamic equilibrium which changes with incoming factors into a complex dynamic equilibrium. Ten percent of muscle protein changes daily, molecule by molecule: in 120 days there can be a complete rebuild of muscle tissue. Muscle is therefore dynamic, capable of being broken down molecule by molecule by protein malnutrition (**catabolism**), and being restructured molecule by molecule by protein synthesis (**anabolism**).

Most muscles are composed of assorted motor units with functional differences, but are dominated by a particular type.

- Tonic muscle fibres (red SO) have a mechanically slow-twitch highly oxidative metabolism. The postural muscles, for example, normally work non-stop except when the body is deeply relaxed (unconscious, paralysed or drunk as a skunk) and require this slow-fatigue status.
- Phasic muscle fibres (white FG) have the mechanically fast-twitch glycolytic (converting glucose to lactate for energy) metabolism, as in the tibial muscles of the lower leg, for sprinting.
- FOG fibres (pink) are mechanically fast with oxidative ability but glycolytic dominance – like the gastrocnemius (calf muscle) for locomotion.

Muscle catabolism (protein malnutrition) occurs through inactivity, abnormality or disorganization: it results in muscle atrophy. In immobilization, for instance, with muscles in their short position, the glycolytic fibres catabolize within 16 hours, and the oxidative in 72 hours (just three days). In the lengthened position entire new sarcomeres are synthesized, adapting to the new longer structure without altering each sarcomere length.

Anabolism occurs with increased activity, and with abnormality or disorganization (such as Duchenne-type muscular dystrophy or with the intake of synthetic derivatives of growth hormones). The result is hypertrophy of muscle tissue.

Muscle fibres are polymorphic, totally adaptable and respond entirely to demand. Their form and function are inter-related – 'FormFunction' in the new language of neuromuscular plasticity, i.e. muscle is subject to exogenous control.

Changing demand is transmitted between muscle tissue and nervous tissue via the terminal synapse (the neuromuscular end-plate), one motor neuron to each motor unit of muscle fibres. End-plates can be:

- rejuvenated as part of a continuing process of transmission;
- replaced;
- re-innervated – a process of 'adoption' by a valid end-plate extending into nearby denervated muscle fibre bundles.

The action potential of an excitable cell such as a neuron is determined by the cell membrane and the changing concentration of ions in the extracellular and intracellular fluid phases it separates. The development of local, graded and non-propagated potentials across cell membranes occurs at synapses between neurons and synapses between neurons and muscle fibres.

The element of uncertainty of response is introduced into the CNS at the neuronal synapses, where the all-or-nothing nature of the action potential is replaced by a dual control of the amplitude of membrane potential change (pre-synaptic inhibition for instance).

The action currents, which are generated by the potential entering the synapse, release molecules of a neurotransmitter from the presynaptic membrane which react with receptor molecules in the postsynaptic membrane. Information is contained in the effected reaction between the molecules of neurotransmitter and the receptor molecules to which they bind.

The changing activity of transmitter molecules and receptor molecules during the procedure of plastic adaptation can be brought about intentionally in clinical rehabilitation. Neurons can be controlled exogenously: absence of demand (exogenous stimulation) leads to a reduction of synthesis with a consequent reduction of ability, and vice versa ('use it or lose it'), i.e. the nervous system is subject to exogenous control. A clear example is the way cardiac muscle responds to consistent exercise training by slowing its pumping rate to enable prolonged activity; this change in rate is controlled by the ability of the CNS to change its output in response to the changing demand upon it.

The control of motor behaviour is cyclic, recursive and plastic.

3.2 PHYSIOLOGICAL STRESSING

All our talents increase in the using, and every faculty, both good and bad, strengthens by exercise.

(Anne Brontë)

Conventional neurology outlined a transient and invariable reaction to the excitatory or inhibitory effect of each stimulus. The 'new' neurology, with the discovery of the plasticity of the neuromuscular system, gives credence to both facultative (having the power to live under different conditions) and enduring changes. Trophic control, by nerve on nerve and skeletal muscle, changes impulse patterns by the release of specific intraneural hormones (neurotrophins) which then act to modify the nervous system so that stimuli can have other effects, i.e. the **brain** is physiologically restructured too.

Of course if a neuronal cell body itself has been destroyed, its restructuring cannot proceed. At cortical level this accounts for the loss of certain specific functions following a stroke, such as hand movement or language construction, and the more general impoverishment of functional activity. No soma = no plasticity, no recovery.

However, impulse traffic can be re-routed by collateral and terminal sprouting and the retrieval or construction of synapses to open up new networks for the surviving neurons. Bach-y-Rita (1981) gives a simple analogy:

> *Let us suppose that the main telephone cables between New York and San Francisco were destroyed in an earthquake. Initially it might be impossible to call from one city to the other. After a time, however, if the demand for this service were sufficient, someone would discover that it was possible to call the telephone operator in Denver, ask that operator to place a call to the operator in Washington, and ask that operator to call New York. This would be effective, but a slow, tedious procedure. Nevertheless, if the demand continued high, the operators at each intermediate city would become more efficient at facilitating the transmission of the telephone information. With sufficient repetition a very high degree of efficiency might eventually be reached that, though less efficient than the original direct line, would very adequately compensate for the loss.*

It is a **system** that is adapting, and not simply a tissue.

Physical activity increases a person's ability to perform physical work (physical performance is quantified in terms of the ability to perform physical work at specific rates and for specific durations). An increasing physical activity can take the form of a therapy that includes a planned component of physical conditioning, which brings about an increase in the capillary density of postural muscles as well as a concomitant adaptation of the enzymes of skeletal muscle. This adaptation of enzyme activity will determine the preferential paths of the metabolism that the muscle will follow as a consequence.

Stressing in the bio-engineering sense is the repetition of a stimulus to produce an analogue effect of faithfully-reproduced stimulation. Receptors are built as required and lost when not required (dendritic growth of the Purkinje cell, end-plate activity, etc.). Physiological stressing is faithful repetition for a significant period of time, to produce change, i.e. frequency and duration of a stimulus.

With new synapses evolving in seven days and strengthened by frequent usage, plastic adaptation occurs in a matter of weeks, not months. The implications for recovery and rehabilitation of stroke are evident: it makes possible the restructuring of normal movement (except where the critical cell is destroyed) but it also builds abnormal motor behaviour – for instance even spasticity becomes self-generating.

3.3 ENABLE OR DISABLE

Any movement, once the critical clinical shock of the impact of a cerebral vascular accident (CVA) has subsided, will have a transient effect on existing systems. If it is repeated then plastic adaptation of the neuromuscular system ensures that it becomes part of the library of motor behaviour for reproduction in all contextual situations. This applies whether the movement is involuntary or volitional, normal or distorted, assisted, resisted or free.

This is where the role of nurses and carers becomes particularly relevant. No matter how effective the episodes of specific therapy intervention, they are only applied at best for short periods in any 24-hour period, other people influence every action performed by the Stroke for the rest of every day, including night-time activity. 'Carry-over' between therapy sessions is dependent upon all the rest of the daily and nightly motor re-learning which takes precedence: a background of greater repetitive frequency and duration creating stronger networks to restructure ability – or disability

An up-to-date appreciation of the facts and the ability to communicate are the only factors involved in this momentous decision – to enable, or to promote the further disablement of, the stroke-survivor. To assist someone to sit and lie in appropriate reflex-inhibiting positions and to move normally is all that is required from non-specialist personnel. Allowing the Stroke to make any movements incorporating the patterns of abnormal posture traditionally associated with stroke rebuilds these abnormalities into every activity. Like spasticity, they become self-generating.

Specialized strategies to unmask and reinforce returning function are outlined in Chapter 10.

3.4 ELECTRICAL NEUROMUSCULAR STIMULATION

A stimulus is anything which produces a response in an excitable tissue. It is also anything assuming the nature of a stressor which modifies, unavoidably, any response by the tissue to further stimulation. Plastic adaptation of muscle is the result of activity, including induced activity from electrical stimulation of the motor point of a muscle (where the motor axons innervate the motor end-plates).

The natural frequency at which a motor unit normally receives action potentials from its motoneuron pool is determined by its role (SO, FG or FOG). Motor units involved in postural control are active more or less continuously: their motoneurons fire at slow rates: 5 to 15 Hz. Other units are activated intermittently and their motoneurons fire at relatively high frequencies.

The mean frequency of the **motor unit action potential** (MUAP) has been derived from detailed analysis of the firing rates of the MUAP of each normal muscle. For instance, slow-twitch skeletal muscle has a mean MUAP frequency of 10 Hz and fast-twitch muscle has a mean frequency of 30 Hz.

It has been shown (Salmons and Vrbova, 1969) in animal studies that when fast muscles are electrically stimulated at low frequencies they become slower to contract and extremely fatigue resistant. Both their biochemical characteristics and their contractile nature are altered by changing the pattern of muscle activity. Their phenotype alters from FG white to SO red: from anaerobic to aerobic metabolism.

Scott *et al.* (1985) demonstrated that similar changes can be electrically induced in human muscles: the selective application of normal MUAP frequencies to muscles deprived of their normal MUAP (as a result of disease, trauma or nervous system impairment) can be used to modify, maintain or restore the gene expression of the muscle fibre.

With knowledge of the recursive factor in neuromuscular adaptation, the clinical implications are awesome.

For paraplegics, the use of selective low-frequency electrical stimulation within carefully proscribed protocols has been shown to reduce persistent severe spasticity to a remarkable degree (Shindo and Jones, 1985). Similar results can be obtained from applying equivalent protocols to 'spastic' musculature following stroke. As in the paraplegic study, the reduction in spasticity can unmask naturally-recovered movement and also allow normal movement patterns to be re-learned (more information about equipment and protocols is given in Chapter 11).

Eutrophic (improving protein synthesis) stimulation of the facial muscles in cases of long-standing facial paralysis (Bell's palsy) using a specifically-designed protocol, demonstrated recovery in all of the designated parameters (Farragher *et al.*, 1987). The atrophied and, in some cases markedly contracted, muscle tissue regained shape and elasticity, and volitional control was re-established.

If a man will begin with certainties, he shall end in doubts, but if he will be content to begin with doubts, he shall end in certainties.

(Francis Bacon)

REFERENCES

Bach-y-Rita, P. (1981) Central nervous system lesions: sprouting and unmasking in rehabilitation. *Arch. Phys. Med. Rehabil.*, **62**, 413–17.

Brown, M.A. and Hardman, V.J. (1987) Plasticity of vertebrate motoneurons, *in Growth and Plasticity of Neural Connections*, (eds W. Winslow and C. McCrohan), Manchester University Press, Manchester, pp. 36–51.

Buller, A.J., Eccles, J.C. and Eccles, R.M. (1960) Differentiation of fast and slow muscles in the cat hind limb. *Journal of Physiology*, **150**, 399–416.

Farragher, D., Kidd, G. and Tallis, R. (1987) Eutrophic electrical stimulation for Bell's palsy. *Clinical Rehabilitation*, **1**, 265–71.

Salmons, S. and Vrbova, G. (1969) The influence of activity on some contractile characteristics of mammalian fast and slow muscles. *Journal of Physiology (London)*, **201**, 535–49.

Scott, O.M., Vrbova, G., Hyde, S.A. and Dubowitz, V. (1985) Effects of low frequency electrical stimulation on normal human tibialis anterior muscle. *Journal of Neurology, Neurosurgery and Psychiatry*, **48**, 774–81.

Shindo, N. and Jones, R. (1985) Reciprocal patterned electrical stimulation of the lower limbs in severe spasticity. *Physiotherapy*, **73**(10), 579–82.

OTHER SOURCE MATERIAL

Kidd, G., Lawes, N. and Musa, I. (1992) *Understanding Neuromuscular Plasticity*, Edward Arnold, Sevenoaks.

Cognition 4

There are no known facts, merely the current theory of the day.
(Carl Popper)

The accurate organization of all human activity depends totally upon the validity of the receiving, processing (decoding and encoding), transmitting and monitoring systems within the higher centres of the CNS. This vital 'processing' is **cognition**.

Cognitive skills are described as being perception, memory and language. The processes involved in 'perception' and 'cognition' are being explored by psychologists, physiologists and neurophysiologists, and by the newly developing professions of neuropsychology and cognitive neuropsychology. Successful functioning in adult life depends upon established cognitive processing – anything else is reflexive or robotic. The following sections, as in all the chapters of this book, need to be read through in sequence so as to build up a better understanding of the relationship between cognition and all functional abilities:

4.1 Perception
4.2 Memory
4.3 Language
4.4 Cognition and motor behaviour – the learning and control of movement

4.1 PERCEPTION

Perception is defined as the ability to interpret sensory messages from the internal and external environment such that the sensation has meaning, i.e. the process is the mental interpretation of a sensory stimulus.

All the incoming signalling requires decoding, organization of the information, and selective encoding of a response – at the higher levels of the CNS – for transmission to the peripheral systems. It is monitored throughout (by ongoing incoming sensory signals) and amended as appropriate for every functional activity: an intact system for processing information.

A successful result is, of course, dependent upon not only the sequential neurological pools of motor engrams (already established networks), but also upon the acquisition of 'rules' and access to memories of previous experiences with which to direct them: the angles of pouring liquids and the sight and/or sound of the rising level in the receptacle, that a sack of potatoes is heavy, that a table is called a table, to stop at the red light, and so on.

For the great majority of people, vision is the primary sensory system, influencing memory, postural responses and the anticipation of movement relative to oneself and to everything else. Examples include: feeding or being fed; avoiding static or moving objects; judgement of two- and three-dimensional space (is it a step or a line?).

For the blind or partially sighted, the tactile, proprioceptive and auditory networks predominate, but for all of us the sensory pathways bring in the information with which to create an organized and catalogued library of experience.

Perception is to do with recognition and previous experience, and the ongoing acquisition of experience in which memory plays the significant role. It is 'a dialectic between self and the external world' (Miller, 1986).

4.2 MEMORY

Memory is the ability to take in, store and retrieve information.

Baddeley (1987) discusses a multiple memory system divided into three categories, broadly based on the length of time for which each stores information:

- sensory;
- immediate;
- long-term.

Information is assumed to be fed into each in turn, from sensory memory through immediate memory into the long-term store.

SENSORY MEMORY

The various sensory systems are thought to be capable of storing sensory information for a very brief period of time. The film industry was so created: cinema film is a series of still pictures in sequence; the image of each is retained just long enough to run into the next to give the illusion of continuous action.

IMMEDIATE OR PRIMARY MEMORY

This is sometimes called 'short-term' memory, but it is an ambiguous term as the length of time involved is only a few seconds. An example of this is looking up a new telephone number and starting to dial it. If you are interrupted or distracted whilst dialling the numbers need to be looked at again. Hitch and Baddeley (Baddeley, 1987) opt for the concept of this immediate memory being a 'working' memory – an alliance of temporary storage systems coordinated by an attentional component labelled 'the central executive'. Of the subsidiary temporary storage systems available to the central executive, the 'articulatory loop', the 'phonological store' and the 'visuospatial sketch pad' are described here.

The **articulatory loop** is a system that utilizes subvocal speech – an 'inner voice' responsible for the speech-like characteristics of many short-term memory tasks, e.g. thinking of a telephone number in words (eight-two-four-five) during dialling rather than in numerals (8245).

The **phonological store** is an 'inner ear' that is independent of articulation, e.g. a fragment of music is not thought of in words.

The **visuospatial sketch pad** is used in creating and manipulating visual images, e.g. recognizing a familiar object when it is presented from an unusual angle.

The **central executive** operates to control functions and allocate resources during task processing.

Rabbitt (1981) and Welford (1980) propose that the decrease in performance found with advancing age may reflect a deterioration in working memory; thus long-term learning can remain unaffected. The more dramatic degradation occurring in Alzheimer's disease, for instance, may represent a breakdown in the central executive, which would severely limit the patient's ability to process information and therefore their ability to cope with the activities of everyday living.

LONG-TERM OR SECONDARY MEMORY

The system of memory responsible for retaining information over a slightly longer time (minutes!) appears to be much the same as that involved in remembering items over a much longer period, but there are distinctions in this too.

Visual and verbal memory

It is possible to remember a particular scene, for instance, in visual terms without needing to think of it in words; or to recognize someone without knowing their name. Conversely there are many instances in which the visual image and the appropriate name seem simultaneously recalled although the visual and verbal processing involved are associated with different areas of the brain.

Episodic and semantic memory

Episodic memory is the autobiographical record, such as remembering what you had for breakfast or the time you nearly got run over some fifteen years ago.

Semantic memory is learned general knowledge on a global scale: wood comes from trees, the name of the American President, etc. Probably great chunks of semantic memory are made up from episodic moments (school bell means end of class), gradually losing the personal aspect with repetition to become 'general' information.

TO SUMMARIZE

'While controversy about the detailed analysis of human memory continues, it can reasonably be divided into three broad subsystems, a set of sensory memories that are grossly related to the perceptual processes and which feed into a working memory system. This is itself quite complex but can be regarded as containing an attentional system (the central executive) aided by a number of subsidiary systems such as the articulatory loop concerned with speech processing, and the visuospatial sketch pad concerned with visual imagery. The working memory system is concerned with the temporary storage of information; as such, it contrasts with the long-term memory system which holds information over much longer periods. Long-term memory in turn can usefully be separated into:

i.   visual and verbal memory, and
ii.   episodic and semantic memory for facts, incidents and events, and
iii. procedural learning – the acquisition of mental and physical skills.

The accurate processing of the memory systems involves the input or learning stage, in which the manner of learning (the degree of attention determining the efficiency) and the ability to catalogue and organize it into a relevant collection of material already held in store; the storage system, and the facility to retrieve it appropriately on demand' (Baddeley, 1987).

4.3 LANGUAGE

Language is the primary means of communicating propositional thought. It is a universal process; every human society has a language, and normal human beings acquire their native language and use it effortlessly. Virtually everyone can master and use an enormously complex linguistic system which depends on sophisticated interaction between sensory-motor skills giving a range of speech sounds, memory and learned syntactic patterns and rules for the organization of speech sounds and words and grammatical sentences.

All languages are composed of a limited number of speech sounds (English has about 40), but the rules for combining these sounds make it possible to produce and understand thousands of words: a vocabulary of 40,000 is not unusual for an educated adult.

Rules for combining words make it possible to produce and understand an almost infinite number of sentences (Atkinson *et al.*, 1990). Sentence units involving strict grammatical rules form the highest level, of skill; words, prefixes and suffixes are the second level; and speech sounds make up the lowest level.

Language is a multilevel system for relating thoughts to speech. It is structured at multiple levels, and the rules enable the combination of units at one level into a vastly greater number of units at the next level.

The speech sounds are formed by the articulators with phonation and resonance to give them accurate identities, which together make words. Learned words make up a lexicon (word store) and are meaningful; many have symbolic association linked to visual, tactile, auditory, olfactory and taste sensations in the memory. A table, snow, bell, buttered toast or skating, for instance, conjure up specific memory-related contexts. Other words serve primarily to make sentences grammatical and so comprehensible.

Language has two aspects: production (expression) and comprehension (reception), both of which involve both spoken and written language.

Broca observed in the 1860s that damage to a specific area on the side of the left frontal lobe of the cerebral cortex was linked to disordered sentence construction and enunciation of words; comprehension of spoken or written language can remain unaffected. In 1874, Wernicke reported that damage in an area of the left temporal lobe resulted in errors in word usage and in the comprehension of both written and spoken language. Geschwind (1979) developed these models further to suggest that Broca's area stores articulatory codes that specify the sequence of muscle actions required to pronounce a word, and that Wernicke's area is where auditory codes and the meanings of words are stored. Spoken words are transmitted from the auditory area to Wernicke's area where the spoken form of the word is matched to its auditory code, which in turn activates the word's meaning. When a written word is presented, it is first registered in the visual area and then relayed on to an area which associates the visual form of the word with its auditory code and meaning.

Much of the earlier work relating speech and language to certain specific parts of the brain is still considered to be applicable. However, it is now recognized that some brain areas may share common mechanisms for producing and understanding speech: for example, when the language areas of the brain are electrically stimulated in the course of a neurosurgical operation, both receptive and expressive functions may be disrupted at a single site.

4.4 COGNITION AND MOTOR BEHAVIOUR – THE LEARNING AND CONTROL OF MOVEMENT

The brain knows nothing of muscles, only of movement.

(F.M.R. Walshe)

The executive role of the CNS in collating cognition and action is well documented, but how it performs this role remains conjectural. The limbic system, for instance, is one which neurologists identify with emotions, memory, motivation, selection and discrimination, taste and smell. 'It probably depends on the setting-up of reverberating circuits – self re-exciting chains of neurons in the appropriate sensory, association and motor areas' (Stein, 1987).

Mulder (1992) introduces his process-oriented model of human motor behaviour with a simple analogy: 'If you observe someone drinking coffee during an interesting discussion, you could see them bending forward while extending an arm to reach for the cup, adapting finger position to its shape prior to grasping it, lifting it carefully to the mouth and then sipping from it. The person stops talking for the sip and the swallow, and then continues; the cup is held for a moment longer somewhere between the mouth and the table, and is then replaced carefully on the saucer. It is an everyday activity – but you are watching a wonderful biological machine designed for adaptive and flexible functioning in an everchanging context – not just a movement but an action with perceptual, cognitive, and sensory/motor elements. Memory provides the knowledge base which is accessed throughout the unfolding motor act.'

Every functional movement is always the result of such a subtle interplay of systems, and requires a fully integrated nervous system. For rehabilitation no one system should be studied out of context. Every movement has intentional aspects and the successful outcome depends on an optimal level of activation. It is probably best represented in Mulder's computational model of motor behaviour (Figure 4.1), which is explained in the following text.

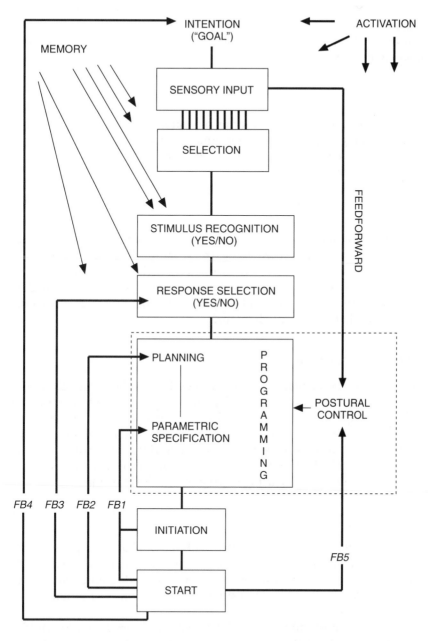

Figure 4.1 Process-oriented model of human motor behaviour. (Reproduced with permission from Mulder, T., A process-oriented model of human motor behaviour, *Physical Therapy* (1991).

ACTIVATION

To perform an act, an optimal level of activation is necessary; extreme exhaustion, coma, alcohol and certain drugs, for instance, lower the arousal level to such a degree that the organism is no longer able to react adequately to stimuli.

INTENTION

Movements should be seen in terms of strategies for solving a problem, or for reaching a goal in the environment (such as picking up a cup of coffee). An intention activates a stored repertoire of acquired abstract motor schemata.

SENSORY INPUT SELECTION

The nervous system is subjected to a continuous bombardment of sensory input, much of which is likely to be irrelevant for the particular act to be performed. Selection of relevant information is therefore crucial to filter out the non-essential stimuli; without this process every bit of data would have the same value and the same potential to trigger a reaction, resulting in chaotic motor behaviour.

STIMULUS RECOGNITION

To determine the relevance of stimuli they have to be identified; this is part of the selection process and dependent upon memory. In drinking coffee, the cup has to be recognized as a graspable object and its significance has to be known. Functional movement cannot be initiated if the stimulus is not recognized – if the telephone rings, only someone who knows it is a telephone ringing will go to answer it. It is necessary to know the context before starting to programme the movement.

RESPONSE SELECTION

The concept of a 'motor programme', with retrieval of a complete unit of pre-programmed muscle response to a stimulus, has been expanded to allow for the subtle interaction between knowledge and movement. Motor learning requires the acquisition of rules, a library of prototypes in more abstract form.

Instead of almost infinite sets of detailed motor programmes, Mulder conceptualizes a limited set of acquired programming rules which together form a 'grammar of action' which functions as the interface between cognition and action. For example, it is possible, without prior practice, to write the same simple phrase with a pen held in the right hand, the left hand, held between the teeth and between the toes; and all of these with the paper close to the body or at a distance (the writing may be shaky, but the words are still written!). Rehabilitation has to incorporate the relearning of all of these motor rules. Repetition of a movement will stimulate new dendritic growth and synapses to supplement or replace impairment, but continued repetition of the movement as a rehabilitation exercise creates only a very narrow prototype which will not enable the recipient to use it in the far wider contexts of normal existence requiring parametric (spatial) specification.

PROGRAMMING

In this model, programming is the construction of *ad hoc* motor programmes on the basis of acquired rules and the actual information selected from the environment. It comprises at least two processes: planning (the ordering and timing of the sequence of operations necessary to perform a required activity) and parametric specification (the adding of context- and task-specific information, such as force and direction, to the motor programme under construction). Disorder in these processes produces ideational dyspraxia and the spatial misinterpretations described in Chapter 5.

POSTURE CONTROL

Perceptual input allows postural mechanisms to be anticipatory, i.e. tuned to future disturbances (as described in Chapter 2).

INITIATION

The sequence of computational processes ends with the actual initiation of the movement.

FEEDBACK (FB) AND FEEDFORWARD

FB1 informs the lower levels of the programme about the selected parameter specifications.

FB2 carries information about the sequencing. Note that planning and parametric errors may occur without affecting response selection; a correctly-selected programming rule may result in a disordered execution because of a planning and/or parametric error, i.e. errors in response selection (the appropriate 'rule' from the library) as demonstrated in ideomotor dyspraxia, can be distinguished from programming errors.

FB3 informs the system about the selected response (rule).

FB4   informs the system about the quality of the task performance in relation to the determined goal: when the goal has been attained the information is stored to increase the existing knowledge base.

FB5   plays a role in the regulation of posture.

The continuous stream of afferent information is needed for the development and updating of the programming rules. Regulation entirely by feedback, however, is often unsatisfactory because the feedback operates only after faulty output has already appeared, so it compensates for disturbances that may no longer be present. Therefore the motor system also operates with a feedforward control mode.

Feedforward   is the sending of some signal ahead of the response in order to prepare the system for input (Mulder, 1991).

This neuropsychological model highlights the complex cognitive and perceptual networking that directs all functional activity. The visible performance of motor tasks cannot be assessed in purely neuromuscular terms.

TO SUMMARIZE

Controlled movement – purposeful and therefore functional activity, and all physical skilfulness and creativity – is initiated and directed by the higher centres of the CNS. Even a little blip will create a chaotic chain reaction, whether the signs are visible or invisible. A stroke strikes at the neurological powerhouse, and no-one survives unscathed. The cognitive and perceptual impairments can devastate a return to independence even when movement appears to be normal.

They are ill discoverers that think there is no land, when they can see nothing but sea.

(Francis Bacon)

REFERENCES

Atkinson, R.L., Atkinson, R.C., Smith, E.E., Bem, D.J. and Hilgard, E.R. (1990) *Introduction to Psychology*, 10th edn, Harcourt Brace Jovanovich, San Diego.

Baddeley, A.D. (1987) Memory theory and memory therapy, in *Clinical Management of Memory Problems*, (eds B. Wilson and N. Moffat), Croom Helm, London, pp. 5–27.

Geschwind, N. (1979) Specialisations of the human brain. *Scientific American*, **241**,180–99.

Miller, N. (1986) *Dyspraxia and its Management*, Croom Helm, London.

Mulder, T. (1991) A process-oriented model of human motor behavior: Toward a theory-based rehabilitation approach. *Physical Therapy*, **71**(2), 157–64.

Rabbitt, P. (1981) Cognitive psychology needs models for changes in perform-ance with old age, in *Attention and Performance IX*, (eds J.B. Long and A.D. Baddeley), Lawrence Erlbaum Associates, Hillsdale NJ.

Stein, J.F. (1987) *An Introduction to Neurophysiology*, Blackwell Scientific Publications, Oxford.

Welford, A.T. (1980) Memory and age: a perspective view, in *New Directions in Memory and Aging*, (eds. L.W. Poon, J.L. Fozard, L.S. Cermac, D. Arenberg and L.W. Thompson), Lawrence Erlbaum Associates, Hillsdale NJ, pp. 1–17.

PART TWO
'Why'

PART TWO

Analysis, assessment and documentation of stroke 5

Go not forth hastily to strive, lest thou know not what to do in the end thereof.

(Old Testament, Book of Proverbs)

All intervention following the stroke, whether medical, surgical or rehabilitative, is based on the assessment of need, which in turn rests on the analysis of the cause of the presenting problems. The actual diagnosis of stroke has to be established: similar signs and symptoms can be presented in many different pathologies (Chapter 11).

A stroke results in brain cell death – this destruction determines the real focal loss incurred, but the scale of this actual loss cannot be accurately assessed for some time after the incident and even then can be difficult to identify. For several weeks after the stroke inflammation and oedema surrounding the site can compress other structures. This is reflected in a greater symptomatic loss initially, which reverses as the acute reaction subsides. Developing spasticity can obscure unimpaired movement, and the plasticity of the nervous system is creating ongoing change and adaptability to activity and handling. All of these factors mask the true facts for some considerable time.

The site of the neural lesion does not always correlate directly with the loss of a specific function (Hertanu *et al.*, 1984). Because the brain is the source and resource organ networking all function, any tissue loss, however small, has an unpredictable effect on human performance. Although many strokes appear to have similarities in effect, no two Strokes can ever be identical in their distribution of disabilities. Moreover, even if the site of the damage as defined on computerized axial tomography (CAT) scans or magnetic resonance imaging (MRI) appears to be the same in two separate cases, the resultant handicaps will be significantly different (CAT and MRI scans are described in Chapter 11). Therefore plotting the site of the lesion on to the traditional 'map' which allots particular functions to specific areas in the brain is of no help at all to the analysis of impairment of function.

Every person has individually constructed and customized networks built from personal experience and endeavour, to say nothing of the pre-natal or genetic differences in the formation of the original structure which allow for the Mozarts, the Leonardo da Vincis, the Charlie Chaplins, right- and left-handedness, dyslexia – and which provide most of us with no extraordinary talents at all, simply individual and often inexplicable little idiosyncrasies. A stroke produces a glitch in this highly intricate and personal mechanism.

Rehabilitation of stroke requires clinical reasoning, defined by Jones and Butler (1991) as the application of knowledge (facts, procedures, concepts and principles) and clinical skills to the evaluation, diagnosis and management of a clinical problem. Clinical reasoning enables problem-solving, the outcome of which determines the success or failure of rehabilitation. Experts appear to be experts not because they solve problems better than non-experts, but because they have a greater store of relevent knowledge and the experience to organize information into meaningful patterns (Grant, 1991).

This chapter explores the collection and organization of information:

5.1 Analysis and assessment
5.2 Analytical assessment
5.3 Predictive assessment
5.4 Documentation in clinical practice
5.5 STARS
5.6 Simple functional mobility chart
5.7 Policy-making
5.8 Audit

5.1 ANALYSIS AND ASSESSMENT

The preceding chapters give the substrata of the idea: the knowledge required for analysis and assessment of the problems that may result from a stroke, i.e. any alteration from the expected normal response to a given stimulus.

ANALYSIS

Assessment and analysis are as interrelated as are form and function. However, in order to develop problem-solving skills it is necessary to understand the problem! Analysis is fundamental to assessment in any dimension.

ASSESSMENT

This can be multidimensional: subjective, objective, quantitative, qualitative, diagnostic, descriptive, general, selective, personal, professional,
perceptive, interpretive or intuitive, sensory, hands-off, hands-on and
comparative.

The assessment of stroke is a perpetual process and multidimensional
for the purpose of rehabilitation. Frames of reference need to be continuously adjusted and readjusted to allow for the changing stroke state.

5.2 ANALYTICAL ASSESSMENT

This incorporates time-related perspectives.

PAST (HISTORICAL)

Impaired-normal or abnormal motor and/or cognitive behaviour is
entirely relative to the subject's pre-morbid (pre-stroke) state.

Details of previous gait and posture, musculo-skeletal status (rupture
of a biceps tendon, a 'frozen' shoulder, arthritic hips and knees, joint
replacements, limb shortening following trauma, and the whole range of
congenital or previously acquired abnormalities); neurological conditions (such as Parkinson's, poliomyelitis, diabetic neuropathies, as well
as earlier strokes); and previous cognitive level must first be elicited from
medical notes and in discussion with the Stroke, family members and
friends, and any other relevent personnel, in order to gain an accurate
picture of post-stroke changes. Family photographs can be very helpful
too.

PRESENT (CURRENT)

This is the presenting motor, sensory and cognitive behaviour following
the stroke. Many therapists work exclusively at this level, which is
perhaps why recovery patterns are often misinterpreted or ignored and
optimal performance may not ever be achieved.

Formal assessment needs to be both specific and comprehensive, and
the preliminaries are important to the accuracy of findings, for example:

- is a hearing aid used or needed? Is it functioning? (learn about hearing aids from an audiologist – and keep spare batteries handy);
- are spectacles needed? Clean the lenses if necessary (very awkward
  for a Stroke who can only use one hand);

- is the Stroke comfortable? (concentration is affected by a full bladder and fear of incontinence or sliding out of the chair);

and so on. Test sensory systems first (impairment affects motor response); details of this are given in Chapter 6.

FUTURE (PREDICTIVE)

This is the expected optimum mobility (the ability to move freely without external aid) relative to the potential to achieve optimal functional capability.

Every treatment episode is designed around continuous assessment of the immediately presenting abilities such as 'that's a promising flicker, let's add this', or the ability to reproduce the response with reduced stimulation, and the evaluation: 'lost it/improved it, try another way'. The responses gained indicate potential ability and future progress.

This predictive analysis should form the baseline for rehabilitation, continuously reviewed against regularly up-dated assessments and relevant to previous ability and changes in environmental or social situation.

5.3 PREDICTIVE ASSESSMENT

There is, as yet, no scientifically-validated or generally-approved system for assessing and scoring outcome. However, as with most situations in everyday life, reading the clues and recognizing the signs gives a surprisingly accurate indication of the next step. Rehabilitation of stroke is a treasure hunt complete with thrills and spills; it requires a map-reader and good teamwork. The usefulness of any evaluation is relative to the level of knowledge and clinical experience of the examiner, and **all** results must be recognized as being 'guesstimated'.

Optimum mobility is dependent upon:

- the degree of actual loss caused by the lesion;
- the concomitant health status (acute or ongoing illness/disease processes);
- multidisciplinary rehabilitative skills.

Potential to achieve optimum mobility is influenced by:

- premorbid status;
- further acute events (of any sort);
- the presence and severity of cognitive dysfunction;
- the presence and extent of acquired reversible disabilities;
- fragmented and/or conflicting rehabilitative techniques.

A very simplistic guide to predictive assessment for use in stroke rehabilitation that depends upon a good understanding of normal human motor/cognitive behaviour and the impairment resulting from stroke (surveyed in the next two chapters) is described at the end of Chapter 10.

5.4 DOCUMENTATION IN CLINICAL PRACTICE

Accurate documentation is important: it provides a relevant and object-ive baseline of information. The need to present a complete written or diagrammatic picture of an individual requires several different forms of documentation, each designed to meet the need-to-know of the different departments involved with the client.

The **medical model** includes medical, surgical and psychiatric history, details of acute episodes requiring intervention, letters and reports of all investigations and examinations, tests and assessments, and notes of all ongoing changes in condition and treatments. These are usually in the form of a patient file, with factual data also on computer, and access to both is limited for ethical reasons. In enlightened hospitals and clinics, profes-sionals other than doctors are also allowed to enter brief details of changes noted, reports on progress and recommendations for management.

Professional models for each discipline record the relevant historical data, a brief account of the acute episode, assessment findings, object-ives, proposed treatment and details of treatment carried out together with dates and times and the subsequent effects, and also accounts of case conferences, family meetings, etc. and the substance of any mean-ingful discussion.

Formal in-depth clinical assessments are usually detailed separately. There are many validated models, only a few of which give the option to record quality of movement. They are all comprehensive and therefore lengthy to work through in a single session – the Stroke can tire quickly, so findings may not be accurate towards the finish – and if the assessment is split then the second half probably won't relate to the first as the picture may well have changed in the meantime! They are inappropriate for frequent clinical use when both time and quiet space are hard to come by.

Problem-oriented medical recording (POMR) is still an excellent method for day-to-day recording, but computerized systems now carry the bulk of data generated, and each system will have its own format for data collection.

Multidisciplinary models attempt to present an holistic record for rehabilitation purposes and ongoing management. It is this form of documentation which is vital to the management of stroke to enable the coordination and monitoring of input and the accurate evaluation of outcome.

Formal assessments need only be carried out infrequently or when requested (for case conferences etc.) because abilities change so rapidly. Initial assessment on first contact is vital; others are needed when activity appears to have reached a plateau or if changes are significant, and a complete assessment prior to discharge or transfer (from hospital or current episode of care) are usually all that are necessary. Careful notes of all intervention and any changes will be recorded in the separate professional records for day-to-day reference.

A survey of both formal and informal documentation models highlights the need for brief but cogent multidisciplinary data-collection and presentation methods. Provided that inter-assessor reliability is established, it is possible to design an informal documentation system that will effectively fulfil local requirements, and which could lead to a formally validated system for wider use. STARS and the simple functional mobility chart are two schemes which have been developed and tested in working situations for use in these circumstances.

'STARS'

The Stow Lodge Assessment and Rehabilitation Scheme was developed by a multidisciplinary team as a structured functional assessment system, and then expanded into a computer-supported database providing an extensive range of sophisticated and colourgraphic information.

The original model, designed for use with the elderly in any setting, is equally applicable to Strokes and other people with functional disabilities. It is a 27 variable ability profile (Figure 5.1) scored 1–4. The current score and a predicted score are entered, and 24-hour activity is monitored, from vision to foot care. It was formulated to bring together the contributions of a dispersed team which had few forums for discussion. The team member of each discipline involved with the client, including night staff, completes their own assessment based on the STARS score sheet. This does **not**, of course, replace specific professional assessments. The team then meets to agree the definitive scores to be formally logged (into the computer if used).

These assessment meetings provide excellent opportunities for team members to gain insight into each other's roles and the client with whom they are working. Training is recommended for these meetings in order to familiarize the participants with the assessment criteria, and also to reassure the timid and those who believe their professional competence is under attack! This is, after all, a general functional ability profile over a 24-hour day, not a statement of what the client can achieve at their best in a session with a specialized professional, and individual scoring may need to be adjusted without prejudice to match the consensus score.

Professional status is **not** a prerequisite for assessors. It may be that in some settings a professional team is unavailable and an identified key

SURNAME _ _ _ _ _ _ _ _ _ _ _ _ _ _ _ _ _   MEDICAL RECORDS No _ _ _ _ _ _ _ _ _ _ _ _

FIRST NAME _ _ _ _ _ _ _ _ _ _ _ _ _ _ _ _ _

STOW LODGE ASSESSMENT REHABILITION SCHEME

ASSESSMENT CRITERIA

ACTIVITY		ABILITY	SCORE	AIM
1	4	Mobile unaided, including stairs and steps		
MOBILITY	3	Mobile with equipment		
	2	Mobile with assistance from people*		
	1	Chairfast		

Comments/Equip _

2	4	Independent		
USING THE	3	Independent with equipment		
TOILET	2	Needs help from people*		
	1	Requires lifting		

Comments/Equip _

3	4	Independent in and out		
IN/OUT	3	In and out with equipment		
OF BED	2	Needs help from people*		
	1	Requires lifting		

Comments/Equip _

4	4	Independent movement in bed		
BED	3	Independent with equipment		
MOBILITY	2	Needs help from people*		
	1	Requires lifting		

Comments/Equip _

5	4	Independent		
TRANSFERS	3	Independent with equipment		
	2	Needs help from people*		
	1	Requires lifting		

Comments/Equip _

6	4	Independent including bathing/strip wash		
WASHING	3	Independent with equipment		
	2	Needs help from people*		
	1	Needs to be washed		

Comments/Equip _

7	4	Independent		
DRESSING	3	Independent with equipment		
	2	Needs help from people*		
	1	Needs to be dressed		

Comments/Equip _

8	4	Feeds independently		
FEEDING	3	Feeds independently with equipment		
	2	Needs help/has difficulty		
	1	Needs to be fed		

Comments/Equip _

Figure 5.1 STARS assessment criteria, numbers 1–8 (of 27). (Reproduced with permission from LHSC Technology, East Suffolk Health Authority.)

assessor has then to refer to other carers who know the client well. In many places the weight of caring is actually in the hands of support workers or family members: their involvement as members of the assessment team has obvious benefits and can spotlight hitherto unseen problem areas, and so promote more realistic appraisal and targeting.

Colour-coded graphs (some clients enjoy doing their own!) or colour-graphic computer print-outs (like figure 5.2, unfortunately here in black and white!) have a dramatic impact as visual aids to the recognition of problem and success areas, to highlighting the need for specific interventions, and to assisting a mixed team (which includes the Stroke) to develop joint goal-setting and to plan joint strategies for ongoing achievement.

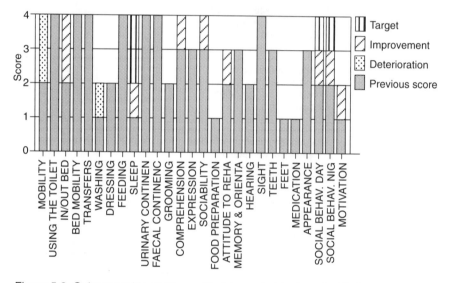

Figure 5.2 Colourgraphic ability profile (shown in black and white). (Reproduced with permission from LHSC Technology, East Suffolk Health Authority.)

With this simple but comprehensive picture it is possible to present a record of each client's functional ability for immediate and comparative use in a number of situations:

- for case conferences, to accompany transfer reports, for progress reviews;
- for client-based provision, development and monitoring of care services (from on-ward nursing care plans to community key workers);
- for advising and counselling with the client and/or relatives and carers.

Computerized individual profiles also assist resource management. For instance aggregated ability profiles in residential settings enable consistent monitoring of on-site activity and quality initiatives – by showing dependency levels, changes in group performance, etc. – and for demonstrating staffing and equipment needs.

These profiles can also assist in the matching and batching of individuals and groups for research programmes, and for comparative studies relating intensity of rehabilitation or different professional techniques to changes in performance, etc.

The system is flexible enough to allow the parameters of this model to be adapted to any requirements; 4 variables scored 1–8, 10 variables scored 1–3 and so on. In conjunction with PAS (Patient Administrative Systems) on IBM-compatible hardware, the STARS computer software can be used to provide a multiplicity of data including standard and enquiry-generated reports, statistics, revenue expenditure and contract monitoring.

5.6 SIMPLE FUNCTIONAL MOBILITY CHART

This simplistic model was designed for multidisciplinary use on a Stroke Unit and to accompany the Stroke into the community setting. The scoring correlated with the Northwick Park Activities of Daily Living Indices scored by the same clients in the occupational therapy assessments – the exceptions being those Strokes with pronounced perceptual impairment (another aid to the recognition of these invisible problems). After a successful pilot study it was adopted for widespread use with Strokes and proved to be equally effective in other areas of work where functional mobility recording is also a problem, in general rehabilitation of the elderly, for example.

Recording general functional mobility within the treatment times available and without losing valuable treatment time has always presented a problem to nurses, therapists and doctors. This model incorporates the everyday moves that reinforce the acquisition of normal activity, and therefore the assessment itself is not only therapeutic but can also be incorporated quite naturally into any other programme or schedule.

Figure 5.3 lists fifteen basic functional mobility requirements for everyday activity, and the criteria for scoring enable it to be applied as a comparative tool in any setting (department, ward, consulting-room, Homes and home) by anyone familiar with it. As in most attempts to record individual performance levels for general use, upper limb function is not specifically recorded; this should feature in the specialized professional assessment models. Safety and competence in everyday mobility is dependent upon dynamic control of movement in relation to gravity, and for this the use of selective S (Stroke-impaired) arm and hand activity is not seen as a prerequisite.

STROKE UNIT MOBILITY CHART

MR-3-692 A.P.

Affix label below if available

Title MR   Surname
Forenames
Address

D of B: 27.1.1911   Age: 82

SCORE:

Total Independence	2
Partial Independence	1
Total Dependence	0
Maximum Score	30

(Verbal OR Physical assistance by one)

(Fifteen movements to Test)

Please Note:

* ROLLING – includes moving across bed prior to Rolling.
* DYNAMIC – includes reaching forwards, up, down and side to side.
* TRANSFERS – includes bed/chair/commode etc.
* WEIGHT TRANSFERENCE – includes Stepping-Through with other Leg.
* WALKING – means safely with stick/frame as required and as normal a gait as possible. State type of Aid if used.

WARD   Side R   Card No.:

No	MOVEMENT	Admission 8.8.92	Date 6.10.92	Date	Discharge 13.12.92
1	* ROLLING to Hemiside	1 P	1 √		2
2	to Normal side	1 P	1 √		2
3	MOVING UP BED	0	0		1 P
4	LYING TO SITTING H. side	1 P	1 √		2
5	SITTING BALANCE STATIC	2	2		2
6	* DYNAMIC	1 P	1 √		2
7	* TRANSFERS	1 P	1 P		2
8	STANDING ⇌ SITTING	0	1 P		2
9	STANDING BALANCE STATIC	0	1 P		2
10	* DYNAMIC	0	0		1 P+Stick
11	* WEIGHT TRANSFERENCE H. Leg	0	0		1 P+Stick
12	to N. Leg	0	0		1 P+Stick
13	* WALKING	0	0		1 P+Stick
14	STAIRS	0	0		1 P
15	UP FROM FLOOR	0	0		1 P
	SCORE	7 / 30	9 / 30	/ 30	23 / 30

Figure 5.3 Simple functional mobility chart.

5.7 POLICY-MAKING

Effective stroke rehabilitation requires special knowledge and seamless teamwork, all of which needs careful organization. This itself requires formal commitment and recognition from every manager and all service providers. Whether the Stroke is admitted to hospital or remains at home, coordinated input is needed and outcomes must be catered for.

Selective admission to stroke unit residential or resource centres should be in accordance with a predetermined policy of needs-testing and assessment by the in-house specialist multidisciplinary team. The formation of a multidisciplinary team is described in Chapter 9.

Ideally a peripatetic multidisciplinary 'flying squad' of specialist professionals should be available in every designated area to advise and monitor those remaining in the community or non-specialist centres, preferably based in the stroke units in order to smooth transition in, out and between. A stroke unit itself requires an operational policy which includes discharge and follow-up procedures.

The following points for reference are taken from the excellent policies written for the stroke unit featured in Figure 9.4 (Chapter 9). The increase in 'length of stay' on the unit, after the initial two year period, resulted from non-adherence to the policies!

ADMISSIONS POLICY

The policy is based upon selective admission.

- selection is by multidisciplinary decision, following formal assessment of each individual case referred in consultation with the team currently managing the patient.
- please refer as soon as possible after diagnosis, ideally within two weeks of onset.
- the patients that will be considered for admission include:
  those who otherwise may not achieve a sufficient independence to return to a community base (own home, suitable rehousing, sheltered accommodation, etc.);
  those who otherwise would not achieve their potential optimum for independence or quality of life after the stroke.
- it will not be appropriate to admit where:
  the patient is medically unstable;
  the patient has other major disabilities which prevent rehabilitation of the stroke;
  recovery is likely to be satisfactory in the existing environment.
- there will be no age-related discrimination.
- the limitation of beds may prevent admission of some patients who fulfil the criteria, however a waiting-list system is not operated (this

could delay or deny the provision of services to those known to be on the list).

Patients may be re-referred.

OPERATIONAL POLICY

- the unit management team includes the medical consultant with overall responsibility for the unit, the nurse-manager, the senior specialist therapists of each discipline involved, the hospital manager and/or the general services manager (or their representatives).
- admission to the unit will be in accordance with the admissions policy.
- all patient management is by multidisciplinary consensus agreement.
- patients who become acutely ill or no longer able to benefit from the services offered on the unit will be referred on and transferred appropriately.
- all discharge decisions will be subject to multidisciplinary team agreement.
- on discharge from the unit, any ongoing rehabilitation needs will be appropriately referred, and continuing contact with the unit will be facilitated.
- the unit has a district responsibility for the pre- and post-graduate education of staff of all disciplines in 'modern stroke management', and is expected to be involved in regional, national and/or international stroke-research projects.

5.8 AUDIT

Audit requires the documentation of systematically and critically gathered evidence about the performance of normal day-to-day practice. Clearly defined purposes and standards need to be set in order to establish the level of performance, to form the baseline from which comparison and evaluation can be undertaken. Clinical audit involves the activities of all health care professionals who work directly with patients or clients. This enables a systematic approach to be undertaken by managers and staff to ensure that quality of service meets expectations and that factors hindering quality provision of care are detected and corrected. It can also indicate the direction towards more desirable outcomes.

Audit is the practical expression of hitherto abstract perceptions such as education, dedication, professionalism and efficiency, and the conscientious search for, research into and application of a means to an end. It cannot, however, replace them – no documentation system could be that comprehensive!

Life is the art of drawing sufficient conclusions from insufficient premises.
(Samuel Butler)

REFERENCES

Grant, R. (1991) Obsolescence or lifelong education: choices and challenges. *Physiotherapy*, **78**(3), 167–71.

Hertanu, J.S., Demopoulos, J.T., Yang, W.C., Calhoun, W.F. and Fenigstein, H.A. (1984) Stroke rehabilitation: correlation and prognostic value of computerised tomography and sequential functional assessments. *Arch. Phys. Med. Rehab.*, **65**, 505.

Jones, M.A. and Butler, D.S. (1991) Clinical reasoning, in *Mobilisation of the Nervous System*, (ed. D.S. Butler), Churchill Livingstone, Edinburgh.

OTHER SOURCE MATERIAL

Lambley, R.F., Darling, R.E. and Smith, D.C. (1990) STARS Research Project, East Suffolk Health Authority and Suffolk County Council Social Services Department, Ipswich.

Abnormal movement and disabled functions

6

'I am a lone lorn creetur,' were Mrs Gummidge's words, ... *'and
everythink goes contrary with me.'*

(Charles Dickens, David Copperfield)

All human beings possess unique differences in their natural skills and
cognitive abilities, and variable competency in functional tasks. Having
explored the established 'norms' of human behaviour and raised awareness of the underlying intricate and infinite biogenesis – in order to
answer the question of 'What is it all about?' – the answers to the following questions should be relatively straightforward:

Why does a stroke produce such a multitude of apparently unconnected
problems?
Why do so many Strokes fail to achieve the standards of performance
expected from rehabilitation?

And, perhaps more to the point,

Why do so many rehabilitation programmes fail to rehabilitate so many
Strokes?

A stroke – a glitch in the central nervous system – produces
immediate disorganization throughout already highly individually
organized systems. It is impossible to relate and collate all the anomalies
(their multiplicity exceeds the studies), but presented here is a selection
of those which are most frequently encountered in clinical practice.
They are divided into **somatic** (motor), **sensory, autonomic,** and **others,**
although the systems are so inter-related and interdependent that
divisions cannot really be justified. Each problem described will be
analysed, but assessment styles are only indicated in the first few
situations for guidance. A rehabilitation principle is indicated where
possible and developed for pragmatic problem-solving in Chapter 10.

Medical and surgical intervention, and medication, are detailed in Chapter 11.

6.1 Balance – postural adjustments to gravity
6.2 Hypotonicity
6.3 Hypertonicity
6.4 Hyper-reflexia
6.5 Spasticity
6.6 Sensory system impairment
6.7 Autonomic system impairment
6.8 Other stroke-related problems
6.9 Depression

[**Cognitive** impairments are described separately, in Chapter 7.]

6.1 BALANCE – POSTURAL ADJUSTMENTS TO GRAVITY

The ability to adjust to gravity is a prerequisite for any movement: it has to be anticipatory, corrective and protective. Balance problems therefore take top priority in stroke rehabilitation.

Balance responses are elicited via the feedback and feedforward mechanisms in the CNS organization of motor behaviour. The effects of disruption in these responses come into three categories: bilateral, unilateral and central. The motor response can be distorted by somatic system derangement, notably that affecting the control of muscle tonus; this is described separately in this chapter.

BILATERAL

Cerebellar and some other brainstem lesions compromise the control and coordination of bilateral movement, characterized by increased postural sway and lurching gait in locomotion (ataxia).

Incoming sensory data, deprived of sophisticated supraspinal control, has to be dealt with at spinal level and produces local alternating stretch–reflex responses at vertebral column sections and the proximal joints. The anticipatory, the programmed corrective elements and the protective reflex mechanisms are still valid, but are shunted into second place giving a slower reaction time – a fall may seem imminent, but is usually aborted.

Strokes with this disturbance complain of 'dizziness' on moving: the vestibular mechanism lacks the fast feedforward and fed-back information necessary to anticipate and adjust to each perturbance, and can only feedback its own disturbance for recognition at cortical level.

Assessment is primarily quantitative: slight, moderate, severe or gross ataxia. Perception is seldom impaired, so a predictive assessment relates to pre-stroke status and post-stroke social and environmental factors.

Rehabilitation uses the Bach-y-Rita principle (practice greatly improves – but does not replace – the lost link).

UNILATERAL

These are usually associated with lesions which primarily affect or destroy sensory neurons or neuronal networks. Tactile and proprioceptive loss on the S side (contralateral to the lesion) knocks out the feedforward of the primary sensory input component and affects the planning and parametric specification (grading of muscle tonus) of the programming and subsequent initiation of postural adjustment. Limb movements on the N side can be initiated and carried out but equilibrium reactions and protective reflex actions are recruited unilaterally, on the N side – the Stroke falls to the S side, often contributing to the fall by increasingly desperate 'bracing' and even pushing by the N limbs in the attempt to regain balance. The problem is common in more severe L strokes (R hemisphere lesions), and can lead to the 'pusher/grabber' syndrome if rehabilitation is delayed or inept.

Assessment is multidimensional, initially for diagnosis and ongoing for evaluation. The predicted outcome is near-normal recovery of balance within a couple of weeks if selective rehabilitation is started early.

Rehabilitation utilizes other sensory and cognitive systems to supplement or replace the reduced or lost sensation, with physiological stressing to re-establish the new networks.

CENTRAL

This is caused by lesions which affect or destroy the programming of postural control, including the serial ordering and grading of postural musculature (Mulder's model, Figure 4.1). Limb movements on the N side cannot be initiated, and protective reflexes are not operational. Sometimes a primitive grasp-reflex is utilized as a protective device, to grab at an immediately adjacent object. This severe disorder usually indicates extensive CNS damage involving many other systems.

Assessment is multidimensional; predictive assessments depend upon the extent of other system involvement. With effective rehabilitation, much of the ability to sustain balance can be restored, but gross perturbations may remain difficult to control.

Rehabilitation utilizes any and every stimulus to recruit a normal response which can, in turn, be incorporated into another – to rebuild the 'programming rules', the grammar of motor behaviour.

6.2 HYPOTONICITY

Apparent paralysis after a stroke is not due to any peripheral nerve involvement, but is the consequence of actual denervation, or disruption in the setting of muscle tonus in the CNS. Where there is focal destruction of upper motor neuron soma, all activity relating to specific muscles or muscle groups can be lost, resulting in a true paralysis and flaccidity. However, in many cases this is a patchy denervation, as only the bundles of muscle fibres enervated by that particular end-plate will be affected; the remaining bundles can be stimulated, but the depleted muscle tissue response may not be strong enough to sustain movement. Joint stability will be affected: the glenohumeral joint is most at risk (Figure 6.1), with the hip coming a close second to give a positive Trendelenburg sign (a lurch to the N side when weightbearing on the S leg).

The repetition of stereotyped reflex activity causes plastic reorganization, which perpetuates the reciprocal grading of antagonist relaxation. With continued disuse the opposing muscle groups catabolize into weakness and apparent flaccidity.

Pat Davies (1990) has identified the major role played by the abdominal muscles in stabilizing the thorax and pelvis in trunk control. With the ever-present underlying hypertonicity of the trunk extensor muscle groups, the opposing flexor groups are consequently at risk from disuse atrophy in addition to a possible direct lesion-related hypotonicity. The resulting floppy tummy is easily recognized – obviously unilateral in many cases – and markedly affects postural control, strength of limb activity, respiration and effective coughing and extra-abdominal pressure.

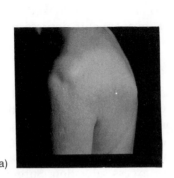
(a)

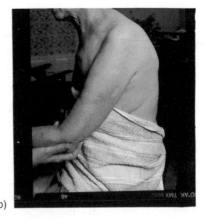
(b)

Figure 6.1 **(a)** Subluxed glenohumeral joint; **(b)** corrected by positioning.

CONTINENCE

Hypotonic abdominal musculature affects the control of extra-abdominal pressure in continence and excretion. Hypotonic detrusor and anorectal musculature leads to impoverished sphincter control, and also the retention of urine and faeces which can result in overflow incontinence. The anorectal angle can also be reduced, allowing continual faecal excretion.

DYSARTHRIA

Hypotonia or flaccidity of the facial and oral musculature is a frequent complication which markedly affects speech and feeding. Accurate phonation, resonance and articulation is dependent upon the variable grading of tone and precision of muscular response. When impaired, the tone and volume of the voice changes or voicing is lost altogether (so that only whispering is possible), and articulation is slurred.

The oral phase of swallowing is inefficient because lips and cheeks – and the tongue in severe cases – cannot give the pressure required to control substances in the mouth, so choking is a major hazard.

Drooling and failing to keep food in the mouth is another frequent and socially-degrading result. Dysarthric Strokes are often undernourished because eating and drinking is such an effort (and embarrassing in the company of others), or seen as greedy because they shovel food into their mouths in copious quantities in order to build up enough pressure (from the incoming food) to push previous mouthfuls backwards to trigger the swallow reflex.

DYSPHAGIA

The complete swallowing mechanism is impoverished or inoperative. The aspiration of solids and liquids into the airways is a major and life-threatening risk, and inadequate nutrition is an often-overlooked consequence in milder cases (fear of choking is a great appetite-depressant).

REHABILITATION OF HYPOTONIC MUSCULATURE

This involves physiological stressing to enhance end-plate activity and to sustain or rebuild muscle tissue. It is directed towards subduing the abnormal reactions, enabling normal reciprocal grading of muscle tone and facilitating functional motor responses. Sophisticated neuromuscular electrical stimulation is very relevant in these instances. Certain drugs can assist detrusor action and reduce excess salivation. Surgery can repair the anorectal angle or brace a glenohumeral joint.

6.3 HYPERTONICITY

The phenomenon of increased muscle tone following CNS lesions is particularly associated with the antigravity musculature concerned in maintaining upright posture – the extensor groups. Decreased supraspinal control increases the excitability of motoneuron pools: the myotatic (stretch) reflex is disturbed by the heightened fusimotor activity, so that sustaining a posture against pressure such as gravity can build up ever-increasing tension in the muscles involved.

TRUNK MUSCULATURE

It is sometimes difficult to differentiate between hypertonicity and hyper - reflexia in these axial muscles. On the whole, hyper-reflexia is more visible in the neck during activity – when the upper fibres of trapezius on the S side spring into prominence – but accurate analysis is less important than effective intervention, which is much the same for both problems. Hypertonicity of the major extensor group of back muscles – erector spinae (sacrospinalis), the lower fibres of trapezius, and quadratus lumborum – can be felt before the increased tone becomes visually noticeable.

Assess by feel. Palpation involving fingertips is often less illuminating than gentle pressure using the whole palmar aspect of the hand against the S side and traversing across to the N side for comparison. In many Strokes, assessed for the first time several weeks post-stroke, the increase in bulk and rigidity of these muscles makes them hugely and visibly prominent (Figure 6.2). At this later stage the tone can be seen building up unilaterally the longer the individual remains standing. The consequential distortion of unilateral extension and lateral flexion to the

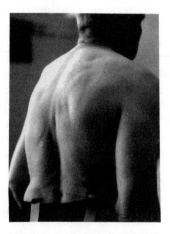

Figure 6.2 Hypertonicity of trunk musculature.

S side accounts for the traditional stroke posture and the inability to correct it to order. The subtle postural adjustments to gravity are lost, directly affecting dynamic balance and fluent limb movement.

LIMBS

Peripheral muscles feel stiff both to the Stroke and to the handler, and a limb will feel resistant to both active and passive movement when compared to the N limb. Remember that normal tone should be low enough to allow effortless movement. Assess S limb movement by gently lifting it – if it feels 'light' (even when muscles are relaxed, normal movement is anticipated and tone adjusted accordingly), then tone is normal. Compare with the N limb (and allow for the initial difficulty that many people have in relaxing!) If all the limbs feel pretty rigid, consider the possibility of underlying Parkinson's disease or post-stroke syndrome.

REHABILITATION OF HYPERTONIC MUSCULATURE

This should either invoke or implement auto-inhibitory systems, and great care should be taken to avoid long periods of static positioning in the erect postures of sitting and standing. Untreated, hypertonia leads to spasticity.

6.4 HYPER-REFLEXIA

When the sophisticated supraspinal control of inhibition and disinhibition is disrupted by stroke, spinal reflex activity is released by the bombardment of sensory stimulation. If these reflex responses are not inhibited, the excitability of the response increases with each repetition (causing neuroplastic changes in synaptic connectivity) until even existing or recovering normal movement is pre-empted by the newly re-programmed hyper-reflexia.

Once established, it is triggered by effort: either involuntarily – such as in sneezing, yawning or coughing – or voluntarily, by attempting purposeful movement or by trying too hard to comply with instructions to move.

The stereotyped reflexes seen in stroke are those of flexion and/or extension of the limbs on the S side, with rotation at the joints which allow it. Other abnormal reflex responses to stimuli are classified by Bobath as static reactions and are defined as follows:

POSITIVE SUPPORTING REACTION (PSR)

This tiptoeing 'push down' response can be elicited by:

- stretching the distal muscles of the limb into dorsiflexion (toes and foot upwards);

- an exteroceptive stimulus (of the sensory nerve endings in the skin) evoked by the contact of the pads of the foot (especially the ball of the foot) with the ground.

The static response ends with the removal of the stimuli.

This reaction makes it impossible to achieve heel strike for normal walking; the S leg either continues into the full extensor pattern so it is held well forwards with marked hip flexion, or it can trigger the flexor withdrawal reflex resulting in a 'bouncing' S leg on attempted weight-bearing.

ASYMMETRICAL TONIC NECK REFLEX

Rotation of the head to one side elicits flexion of the arm on the opposite side, and extension of the arm on the side to which the head is turned (Figure 6.3). In severe cases it is impossible even to convey food to the mouth. In a milder form the head is kept turned to the preferred N side and is strongly returned to face that side when any activity is attempted. This is enhanced by walking with one stick using the N arm, which involves extending the arm on that side; the S arm is then further reflexed into the flexed position even when normal movement patterns are present.

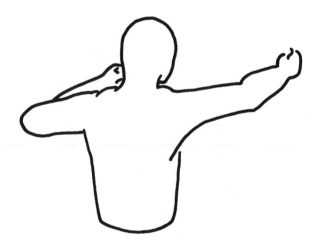

Figure 6.3 Asymmetrical tonic neck reflex.

SYMMETRICAL TONIC NECK REFLEX

Forward flexion of the neck triggers flexion of both upper limbs with extension of both lower limbs; neck extension extends the upper limbs and flexes the lower limbs. The patterns can be easily identified in domestic cats: watching something above it, the cat sits down with fore-limbs braced and head raised back; when a cat lowers its head to drink from a saucer of milk, the front legs flex and the hind limbs extend. This is often a feature of central lesion Strokes who despite useful bilateral limb movement appear to 'fold up' when attempting to walk. As they brace their legs for initial standing, the upper trunk and arms are irresist-ably drawn into flexion – given assistance on each side they appear to dangle between their helpers and eventually a full flexor-withdrawal reflex can be elicited in the lower limbs also. When pushing up from a chair – or given a walking frame once up, when the reverse situation is exposed – on bracing the arms in an attempt to straighten up, the legs buckle into flexion; on extending the legs, the arms bend and the upper torso tips forward (Figure 6.4).

REHABILITATION OF HYPER-REFLEXIA

This relies on selective and dynamic fragmentation of the reflex patterns. Untreated, hyper-reflexia becomes hard-wired into spasticity.

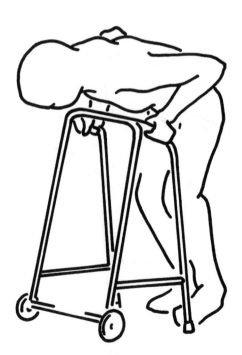

Figure 6.4 Symmetrical tonic neck reflex.

6.5 SPASTICITY

Spasticity does not occur immediately following the stroke, but results from the neuromuscular reprogramming of:

- sustained hypertonicity;
- frequently activated stereotyped reflex patterns;
- hyper-reflexia.

It can be painful and makes movement abnormal and exhausting.

Spasticity is increased by persistent non-weightbearing through the S side (neglecting the secondary peripheral system of presynaptic inhibition). It distorts existing normal movement and obscures – or prevents the use of – recovering normal movement.

Persistent over-use of the N side (limbs and trunk) in compensatory attitudes can result in hypertonia and sometimes spasticity of this hitherto unaffected side of the body as well.

Clinically, spasticity presents as:

- increased resistance to passive movement of the limbs; they feel heavy and stiff to the Stroke and to the handler, and the range of joint movement can be markedly reduced (this needs to be compared with movement on the N side to eliminate arthritic changes, for instance). When testing the S arm ensure that the **whole** shoulder girdle – including the scapula – is moving normally, to prevent trauma at the glenohumeral joint.
- gross non-functional movements in the stereotyped reflex patterns in response to stimulation or activity.
- inappropriate co-contraction of muscle groups (instead of graded reciprocal activation).
- inability to fractionate patterns to perform selective movement.

Spasticity is not confined to the S limbs. The **trunk** musculature is affected even in mild strokes. Spasticity of the muscles supporting the vertical body on the S side accounts for the traditional posture and a sidling gait: the shoulder girdle is retracted backwards and downwards and the pelvis is drawn up and rotated backwards (Figure 6.5). In standing this creates flexion at the S hip and the apparent shortening of the S leg, e.g. standing and/or walking with the N knee slightly flexed (Figure 6.6) is a sign of compensatory response.

Spasticity of the trunk musculature is the major – yet frequently unrecognized – source of both continuing and progressively worsening physical disablement of stroke survivors. Unchecked, the integral stability of normal postural control (which depends on continuous adjustment to gravity for balance and the effortless initiation of limb movement) is destroyed. A totally valid sense of insecurity over-rides all dynamic

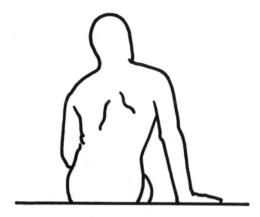

Figure 6.5 Sitting posture distorted by stereotyped reflexes.

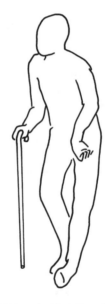

Figure 6.6 Compensatory posture in standing: S arm in the 'waiter's tip' reflex position.

mobility, and this anxiety, with the effort involved in the production of movement, generates increased hypertonia, reflex activity and spasticity.

Rehabilitation is directed at restoring self-inhibitory mechanisms.

Other systems can be severely affected by hypertonic and spastic musculature too.

CHEWING, SWALLOWING AND SPEECH

Lip contour and lip movement is minimized, affecting salivatory and substance containment (causing dribbling and drooling). The whole tongue can be contracted and cannot be extruded, or, with unilateral contraction, it is deviated to the S side. Manipulation of the food bolus is difficult or impossible and liquids cannot be controlled, therefore the preparatory and oral phases of the normal swallow mechanism are jeopardized. Articulation is severely affected.

Rehabilitation utilizes every trick in the trade to inhibit spasticity except the application of ice to the muscles of and surrounding the lips, which is thought to endanger cardiac function (Chapter 8).

VOIDING AND EXCRETION

Failure of CNS inhibition of the monophasic reflex arc leads to involuntary contraction of the detrusor muscles in response to the filling bladder, resulting in urinary incontinence.

Constipation leading to impaction of faeces can result from spasticity of the anorectal musculature, so the cause needs to be identified. Untreated, it can present as diarrhoea (overflow faecal incontinence). Poor diet and lack of exercise can be contributory factors.

Anti-spasticity agents can help to reduce severe spasticity, but the side-effects often create other problems.

Rehabilitation is discussed in Chapter 10.

6.6 SENSORY SYSTEM IMPAIRMENT

The reception and the processing of all sensory input can be disturbed by a stroke. Tactile and proprioceptive information is most at risk, but vision, hearing, taste and smell can all be affected.

Sensory loss or impairment can jeopardize personal safety and compromise feeding and articulation. Impaired reception of sensory data from the bladder and anorectal structures results in reflex incontinence. Motor programmes can remain uninitiated, and the speed and accuracy of movement is greatly reduced. Weight-transference and walking demand exceptional courage and perseverance – the transference of body-weight, to a limb that 'isn't there' because no sensation from it is being recorded, is naturally rejected by the cognitive executive system. Re-learning is more difficult: neuromuscular plasticity depending upon responses to sensory stimuli is impoverished.

Impaired or lost tactile and proprioceptive sensation is a feature more associated with lesions in the right hemisphere, (L strokes).

Hypersensitivity can result in misery and, in a few cases, severe pain. Left hemisphere lesions (R strokes) show a higher incidence of hypersensitivity, and visual disturbances are more common, ranging from generally-impaired focusing to hemianopia and tunnel vision.

Simple testing is necessary to assess the extent and degree of sensory loss on the S side, with matched testing of the N side for comparative purposes.

TACTILE

The responses to light stimulation on the skin are tested in 'spot' checks – stimulating larger areas can cause confused responses. Certain areas are more sensitive than others – try touching your nose with a fingertip: the sensation from the nose takes precedence over that from the fingertip.

Test with: fluffy cotton-wool, single fingertip pressure (light touch and a deeper 'prod'), sterile disposable 'pinprick' points and a warm and a cold article (test-tubes of water, for instance).

Clear instructions need to be given, including, 'Tell me **when** you feel this', 'What does it feel like?' The subject should not be watching: wincing at the pinprick test could be inspired by previous experience (and some Strokes don't like to feel they are depriving their assessors of an expected response!).

Test first the superficial skin sensation.

Continue to test, particularly if this is deficient, for:

- **Two-point discrimination** equal feeling at both points when the same test is applied simultaneously to two points in the same area.
- **Bilateral discrimination** equal feeling at both points, when the same test is applied simultaneously to the same point on the S and the N limb. It is possible for recognition of the stimulus on the S limb to be 'obliterated' by the stronger reception of sensation on the N side; this is more common in Strokes who also display unilateral neglect (Chapter 7).

PROPRIOCEPTION

Again, testing is done with the subject's eyes closed to prevent visual clues. Limbs are passively moved through a small range, then a larger range, and the person is asked, 'What position is your knee in now?' (bent, straight, bending more, etc.), 'Is your hand palm up or down? Is your finger moving? Which finger?' and so on.

VISION

Various anomalies can occur in the visual fields, due in many instances to impaired control of the eye musculature as well as impairment of the reception and processing of sensory information.

The problem of recognition of objects is a cognitive disorder and is described in Chapter 7.

Hemianopia is defective vision or blindness in half of the visual field of one or both eyes. A lesion in one hemisphere of the brain can destroy the reception of input from the contralateral side of the visual fields.

Homonymous hemianopia is hemianopia affecting the right halves or the left halves of the visual fields of both eyes.

HEARING

This can be altered by a stroke. Usually unilateral, it is often misdiagnosed as a defect in the auditory mechanism – or disregarded. The effect is a reduction or 'muffling' in the reception of sound, and occasionally tinnitus.

TASTE AND SMELL

Another infrequent impairment following stroke, this can be related to dysarthric problems.

'THALAMIC PAIN'

This is an extension (in some two percent of strokes) of the hypersensitivity associated with left-hemisphere lesions, and can affect all or part of the S side of the body. It is described as 'burning', 'shooting', 'throbbing' or just 'terrible', and seems to be similar to the neuralgia that can follow *herpes zoster* infection (shingles). Sensation in the painful area is often abnormally heightened, but the presence or absence of touch sensation seems to be irrelevant to the degree of pain experienced. Oddly, the pain does not appear to disturb sleep and this is often the only respite. This pain syndrome was first detailed in 1906 by Déjerine and Roussy in three subjects with thalamic lesions; however it is now accepted that the thalamus is affected in only a minority of cases. The sympathetic tracts of the autonomic nervous system are always involved, so that skin temperature in the pain area is lower than at the same site on the other side even when 'burning' sensations are reported, and the skin sometimes feels sweaty or clammy.

Post-stroke thalamic pain may occur immediately, but more usually develops much later. It can be severe, and conventional pain-blockers, whether chemical or electrical, are ineffective. Surgical intervention is at present an experimental and expensive last resort which can be very effective (Chapter 11).

REHABILITATION

For sensory system impairment this includes a whole battery of sensory-stimulating (or reducing, in the case of hypersensitivity) techniques, but most sensory losses are irreversible, from focal destruction. Any recovery is usually fairly early post-stroke after the acute inflammatory reaction has subsided or due to natural repair. Teach the Stroke to utilize the remaining and intact sensory systems by, for example, looking to check position of S limbs and environmental hazards, feeling with the N hand and foot to locate S limbs.

6.7 AUTONOMIC SYSTEM IMPAIRMENT

There seems to be a dearth of information about the effect of stroke on the autonomic system.

The 'shoulder-hand' syndrome discussed in the next section is likely to be the result of poor autonomic control of the circulatory system musculature, compounded by hypotonic and therefore unsupportive somatic musculature. The same effect is seen peripherally in both upper and lower limbs – producing oedema and white/mauve/purple/blue (depending upon the position in relation to gravity) blotchy and clammy skin. The gross 'cold' oedema of a S limb (usually the S leg) could also be attributed to autonomic impairment. These are discussed further in section 6.8.

There is definitely an associated, although mechanically-induced, effect in relation to posture (Chapter 2). The 'slump' position already described elongates the spinal cord and peripheral nerves causing undue stretching – and therefore narrowing – of the feeder blood vessels within the nerves. This impoverishes the innervation of the somatic musculature and contributes to the catabolic degeneration of muscle tissue.

The often severe abdominal pain, distension and 'windiness' that is a problem for many Strokes in the early stages is probably due to hypotonic somatic abdominal musculature directly affecting extra-abdominal pressure, but impoverished peristalsis in the viscera could also be a contributory factor.

Excess production of saliva is another autonomic system blip.

Rehabilitation concentrates on activity to raise tone in the somatic muscles and to improve circulation, positioning to prevent gravitational oedema and drooling, and careful monitoring of all sitting postures, particularly for people who are likely to spend all day slumped, awake or asleep, in semi-reclined chairs, chin on chest, legs outstretched on floor or stool, with arms dangling.

6.8 OTHER STROKE-RELATED PROBLEMS

DENTURES (AND MOUTH)

If dentures remain unworn for a period of time – while a Stroke is coma-
tose, for instance – then gum shrinkage occurs and false teeth no longer
fit. Regular gentle brushing (as for teeth) will maintain gum bulk until
the dentures are in use again.

With hypertonia or hypotonia of the facial musculature, dentures are
difficult to keep in place. Both factors affect competency in speech and in
eating, and therefore need to be addressed as soon as possible. Dental
fixative can be a useful interim measure, but new dentures may be needed.
In these circumstances some dentists will do home visits if necessary.

Flaccid cheeks can get bitten or chewed on the inside: warn of, and
watch for, mouth ulcers. With sensory loss, pieces of food (sometimes
huge!) can get pocketed in the cheek and cause infection; fingertip-search
and rescue after every meal, until the Stroke is able to do so independently.

DIZZINESS

Fluctuations in blood pressure often present management problems:
postural hypotension (low blood pressure) is a fairly common hazard,
particularly when starting to mobilize Strokes who have been on bed
rest for a while. These individuals will feel faint or dizzy on coming
upright or on standing for too long. Proceed gently and arrange for
blood pressure checks in lying and standing positions. If the problem
does not resolve itself naturally fairly quickly, medication will need
to be reviewed.

Elderly people are more susceptible to medication than their younger
counterparts (and are frequently receiving more). Sedatives and general
muscle relaxants in particular can create a sense of 'muzziness' in many
older clients. Review medication.

Ongoing problems not caused by low blood pressure or drugs are
often associated with brainstem lesions and ataxia. Many Strokes experience dizziness or giddiness during waking hours, usually exacerbated
by movement. Possibly this is due to disruption in the processing of
vestibular signals: every miniscule slosh in the semicircular canals being
registered instead of being translated into motor behaviour programmes.
Some of these Strokes feel nauseated, too, and can suffer severe travel
sickness post-stroke (sitting sideways to forward motion, as in some
ambulance vehicles, can be particularly upsetting).

Conversely, Camillo Azzopardi, who features in the photograph at the front of the book, suffers from continual dizziness when he is moving in relation to a fixed base – which is all the time he is walking, standing and working or sitting. Only lying down gives respite – and, interestingly, so does driving his car or his horse-drawn trotting rig. For him, movement in relation to a secure but randomly moving base (i.e. subjected to external perturbation) seems to stimulate or jump-start the normal processing.

DROOLING

Associated with dysarthria and with facial muscle hypotonia, it may also result from lost sensation within and around the mouth so that the presence of normal saliva is unnoticed until it collects and over-flows. It can also indicate an autonomic system disturbance causing over-production of saliva; this may be moderated with appropriate medication.

Rehabilitation includes teaching postural control of head and neck, with lip closure and swallowing re-education. Protect against likely soreness at the corner of the mouth with appropriate ointment, in the meantime.

EMOTIONAL LIABILITY

This presents as inappropriate – or appropriate but excessive – crying or laughing. To distinguish it from the purely psychological state (which is unconnected with actual brain cell trauma) it is now being renamed as **emotionalism**, and is often associated with lesions causing dysarthria and dysphagia. It causes embarrassment and distress, particularly to carers, and the copious weeping is often mistaken for a depressive state. It has nothing to do with depression, however, nor with perception, although it is commonly listed among the perceptual problems.

Treatment is simple at present: disregard the outbursts as tactfully as possible (offer a handkerchief when appropriate) and don't reinforce by consoling the tears or promoting the laughter: this will exacerbate it. Reassure and advise all concerned to 'carry on regardless'. The frequency tends to diminish as time goes on.

EPILEPSY/FITS

These can occur in some 10–15% of cases, usually starting some months after the stroke (possibly due to residual cortical scarring) and continuing haphazardly for two or more years. These fits, whether major or minor, do not seem to occasion further damage; in certain instances a fit has resulted in an apparent clearing of obstruction and the actual recovery of a piece of the cognitive jigsaw.

In one case study, a Stroke with severe dysphasia which included complete loss of numeracy had been subject to several fits over a period of eighteen months. After one particularly severe grand-mal attack he was re-assessed as usual and was found to have recovered basic numeracy skills. The treatment is simply medicinal – by prescribed drugs for the epileptic condition. A UK driving licence cannot be re-authorized until two full years have elapsed without a fit.

INCONTINENCE

This frequently features in the acute post-stroke phase, but should respond quickly to conservative measures as an integral part of the normal recovery process. Apparent faecal incontinence can develop as a result of constipation or faecal impaction which leads to overflow.

Reassurance and regular and frequent assisted toiletting, and progressive mobilization which serves to readjust muscle tone and activity, are an important part of the rehabilitation programme. Medication and electrical neuromuscular stimulation (described in Chapter 3) have been discussed earlier in this chapter and are detailed in Chapter 11.

In very few cases of severe stroke damage incontinence remains a problem and then requires invasive intervention such as catheterization.

OEDEMA/SWELLING

Oedema in dependent or dangling limbs results from a combination of hypotonic musculature, autonomic system impairment, and/or decreased mobility and gravity. This should respond to movement, careful positioning and light elasticated supports if necessary.

A gross 'cold' oedema of an entire limb – usually the S leg – is an occasional post-stroke complication, probably due to autonomic system involvement. Pressure bandaging and 'flowtron' treatment (with caution) can reduce the severity, but a permanent pressure garment will be required in most cases to maintain adequate control (there are hints on easy application in Chapter 13).

Oedema around a joint – usually the S ankle – is due to trauma. Warm and flushed indicates acute sprain or inflammatory response to sustained pressure (just before skin breakdown). Cold and blotchy implies chronic repetitive trauma. Treat accordingly, and prevent recurrence.

PAINFUL JOINTS

These can develop as a result of autonomic (sympathetic) system involvement, and a local inflammatory reaction produces gout symptoms, particularly in the fingers and carpo-metacarpal joints.

Pain is also a result of prolonged abnormal posture and limb patterns, in both activity and inactivity, causing soft-tissue trauma and eventual joint damage. Many Strokes are referred for orthopaedic intervention or physiotherapy for 'sciatica', 'back-pain' or 'frozen shoulder', which on analysis prove to be rooted in chronic post-stroke hypertonia and acquired trauma or disablement. For rehabilitation see the next section.

PAINFUL SHOULDER

This is **not** a natural phenomenon of stroke, it is the result of acquired trauma. Hypertonicity/spasticity preventing free shoulder-girdle movement, hyper-reflexia, and hypotonicity which leaves the glenohumeral joint unsupported and unprotected, all contribute to the extreme vulnerability of the glenohumeral joint and its soft-tissue structures to external forces. The gravitational subluxation (a 'pulling apart') due to lack of support by hypotonic musculature can be relatively pain-free (even when sensation is unimpaired) until the joint is abused.

Careless lifting and handling by others, as well as self-inflicted injury due to enthusiastic compliance with 'DIY' exercises, cause most of the damage. With hypotonia the glenohumeral joint is frequently dislocated and is easily displaced; the head of the humerus is often found to be wedged forwards, under the clavicle.

Strong hyper-reflexia in opposing patterns such as the 'waiter's tip' – where the pectoral muscles inserting into the humerus pull the arm up and forwards across the front of the chest and extend and medially rotate the elbow – in conjunction with the ever-present extensor pull of the back muscles which drag the scapula down and backwards, can also dislocate the joint.

Pain is the normal consequence of damage to the soft tissues (ligaments, tendons, capsule) of this joint.

Rehabilitation is primarily preventative. Prevent trauma in the first instance, and intervene to correct ongoing traumatic procedures. Second it is alleviative, to reduce pain and to assist healing of the damaged tissues.

PARKINSONIAN TRAITS

Seen in some central and brainstem lesions, these present as a symmetrical facial rigidity or lack of facial expression, with bilateral impairment of movement initiation and fluency (not to be confused with the dyspraxias of movement which are detailed in Chapter 7). This usually responds well to minimal doses of certain drugs prescribed for the treatment of Parkinson's disease.

SHOULDER-HAND SYNDROME

This is associated with somatic hypotonia and possibly autonomic system impairment. The stroke hand in particular feels 'clammy' and cold to the touch, looks white, pink, mauve or blue and swollen according to its position in relation to gravity (resting horizontally or dangling down).

The musculature of the stroke arm, shoulder and neck on the stroke side is flaccid allowing the glenohumeral joint to distract (pull apart). The circulation and nerve supply to the arm could be impaired as a result of the gravitational down-pull of the arm overstretching these tissues, but this factor is probably only compounding an existing sympathetic involvement.

Management includes the provision of adequate support to the stroke arm and hand which will also re-align the glenohumeral joint, and measures to regain tone in the hypotonic muscles.

SOFT-TISSUE CONTRACTIONS

These can be apparent or real. 'Contraction' of muscles and tendons may just be the spastic reflex patterning of limb postures, which respond to reflex-inhibitory procedures. If some shortening has resulted from long-term abnormal positioning, then it is worth using electrical neuromuscular stimulation protocols which re-establish the trophic code. For severe shortening, careful serial splinting may be necessary to encourage the growth of new sarcomeres.

Really long-term inactivity can of course deplete bone integrity, resulting in osteoporotic changes. If this is suspected, the joints in question need to be X-rayed before any attempts are made to increase range of movement.

6.9 DEPRESSION

The depression suffered by Strokes is unlikely to be a 'clinical' depression, but is a natural and non-permanent reaction to any arbitrary change in life circumstance. The degree of depression varies with the individual's own perception of their situation and their pre-stroke coping skills. Their partners suffer too, and often for longer, as they bear the brunt of decision-making and the prospect of ongoing responsibility and role changes.

NATURAL DEPRESSION

Natural depression is compounded of anxiety and grieving.

Anxiety can be allayed firstly by careful and appropriate explanation of the stroke itself and the particular problems concerned in each case, giving plenty of reassurance and room for optimism as to future improvements. Be prepared to repeat all this as often as it seems to be required.

Every Stroke will improve – it is only the degree of improvement that is unforeseeable. Far too many people give time limits to this when talking to the family (and to the Stroke, too). **There is no time limit to recovery after stroke**. Describe 'neuromuscular plasticity' and convey this as often as necessary in all conversations. Progressive achievement in itself will boost morale: a video camera is useful (see Chapter 10) to record individual progress which can be replayed to the person – and to their family and friends, too, with due approval – when they feel downhearted.

Grieving lasts longer. Stroke is a form of bereavement and it can sometimes take one to two years to come to terms with the loss of pre-stroke normality, and to accept the altered self-image, changes in lifestyle and probable readjustments in family relationships. Worden (1986) and others list the manifestations of normal grief as:

- feelings   –   of sadness, anger, blame (blaming oneself or others for the loss), guilt and self-reproach, anxiety, loneliness, feeling different or somehow alien, fatigue, helplessness, shock, and yearning;
- cognitions   –   disbelief, confusion, preoccupation, hallucinations or a sense of 'presence' (of that which has been lost);
- behaviours –   sleep disturbances, appetite disturbances, absentmindedness, social withdrawal, restless over-activity and crying.

These manifestations of normal grief, after the death of a loved one, encompass some if not all of the reactions experienced by anyone suffering with physical and mental illnesses too. We need to be aware of these in order to understand better the misery felt by those we are trying to rehabilitate, and their families, too; their bereavement also needs to be rehabilitated. Worden (1986) describes four main tasks of mourning (the amendments in brackets relate it to stroke):

- to accept the reality of the loss;
- to experience the pain of grief;
- to adjust to an environment in which the deceased (previously normal ability) is missing;
- to withdraw emotional energy and reinvest it in other relationships and activities.

Parkes (1972) also names four phases of mourning; three to be worked through:

- numbness;
- yearning;
- disorganization and despair;

to reach the fourth: reorganized behaviour.

These tasks need to be completed as part of the rehabilitation process in order to regain any quality of life. As an informal guide, the goals need to correspond to the tasks, and Worden advises counselling to:

- increase the reality of the loss;
- help the bereaved deal with the expressed and latent effect;
- help the bereaved to make a healthy emotional withdrawal from the deceased (past);
- and to feel comfortable reinvesting that emotion in the substitute (present and future life).

Some people have great difficulty in readjusting to life after a stroke, and it may be helpful to introduce them to more expert guidance. In these circumstances a family bereavement counselling service – with a counsellor who can relate bereavement to disability – is sometimes more constructive than that offered by a non-neuropsychology service, which may see this 'depression' in purely behavioural terms. For the Stroke and family too, referral to a psychologist may add to the anxiety: the difference between psychology and psychiatry is seldom clearly understood, and any misunderstanding could further upset even the most rational person's view of the situation.

It is important also to remember that emotionalism following stroke is not to be confused with depression, although it can of course be enhanced by the loss of 'normality'. If this factor is significant, it needs to be recognized and handled appropriately.

Depression is a symptom in some debilitating diseases; anxiety is a symptom in many endocrine disorders and also the result of unstaged drug withdrawal (from Valium, for example).

The side effects of medication can also produce depression and anxiety (certain anti-hypertensives for instance), and lethargy (which is often a sign of depression); these are described in Chapter 12.

CLINICAL DEPRESSION

This is an entirely different state, and if any person has a history of depression pre-stroke – or whose reaction of natural depression following the stroke seems unnaturally severe, or long-lasting, or worsening – then they require psychiatric help. Excessive anxiety, depression or anger, undue fatigue, lethargy, weight-loss, headaches and disturbed behaviour without clinical cause, are all symptomatic of a clinical depression.

> For five months I have been on a plateau of misery ... a kind of alone-ness is with me now. I have to curl up deep inside myself. For the moment I have no energy (even for the telephone)...
>
>   I have reached again a hard place in my illnesses. I am on the edge of anger all the time ... Lonely, desperately when no one is here, and then exhausted if anyone is ...
>
>   ... I feel I have lost control of my life, look forward to nothing, live the days through like a zombie, (and long for sleep, oblivion)...

... I can no longer 'respond' as I used to ... I feel so cut off from what was once a self ...

That was how the writer May Sarton felt on her depression, following a stroke.

If the brain were so simple that we could understand it, we would be so simple that we couldn't.

(Emerson Pugh)

REFERENCES

Davies, P. (1990) *Right in the Middle: selective trunk activity in the treatment of adult hemiplegia*, Springer-Verlag, Berlin.
Parkes, C.M. (1972) *Bereavement: studies of grief in adult life*, International Universities Press, New York.
Sarton, M. (1988) *After the Stroke: a journal*, The Women's Press, London.
Worden, J.W. (1986) *Grief Counselling and Grief Therapy*, 2nd edn, Tavistock Publications, London and Springer, New York.

Cognitive impairments

7

He that hath no rule over his own spirit is like a city that is broken down, and without walls.

(Old Testament)

Many of the problems affecting stroke survivors seem to relate clearly to either the 'dominant' hemisphere (which will contain the language processing area) or the 'non-dominant' hemisphere (which controls much of the 'common-sense' processing) of the brain. In the majority of humans the dominant half of the brain is the left hemisphere, giving right-handed skills dominance over the left-handed ones.

Normal functional activity, however, is the result of complex conceptual activity, and requires integrated and coordinated working of **both** cerebral hemispheres. Lesions in right or left hemispheres can cause visible problems in the contralateral side of the body, but they also cause an infinite variety of complex invisible problems which are often misunderstood and simplistically misdiagnosed as confusion, dementia, psychosomatic and behavioural or personality disorders (such as wilful refusal to comply with rehabilitation strategies!).

In fact the pre-stroke level of intelligence is unaffected, but the ability to use it competently may be devastated: this renders the sufferer puzzled, frustrated and increasingly depressed – and can stress everyone else beyond belief.

'Lack of motivation' is the phrase frequently used to label many Strokes who fail to achieve the expectations of professional and domestic carers alike. In fact this is usually a failure by these significant others to recognize the complex cognitive dysfunction – in memory, perception or language, together with its effect on the organization of motor behaviour and communication skills – underlying the visible disabilities. The result of this lack of awareness is non-effective rehabilitation with consequent despair and eventual apathy in the recipient (probably mirrored in the professional and family carers, too).

7.1 Memory
7.2 Perception/cognition
7.3 Apraxia/dyspraxia
7.4 Unilateral neglect
7.5 Language

7.1 MEMORY

All the memory systems described in Chapter 4 are vulnerable, and any part of them can be erased or rendered inaccessible by the stroke lesion. Most of the 'perceptual' problems are memory-related.

Formal assessment is helpful for the analysis of associated deficits in performance; informal assessment can be noted in relation to the activities of daily living.

There is no evidence yet that memory can be rehabilitated. Repetitive tasks that relay lost or impaired motor skills do not improve memory. It is necessary instead to utilize intact relearning ability or to teach strategies that can circumvent, compensate or supplement the original process.

7.2 PERCEPTION/COGNITION

Listed and defined here are some of the identified perceptual problems that may occur following stroke. They are gathered alphabetically into the major groups for easier referencing. The three which generally cause the most obvious disruption to the restoration of functional status in everyday activities are dyspraxia, unilateral neglect and aphasia. These are discussed in more detail later. Note that the prefix 'a' means total loss of, while the prefix 'dys' denotes partial loss or impairment. The list contains both forms, somewhat haphazardly, as they are in common usage, and includes a few disorders which are sometimes described as 'personality changes'.

AGNOSIA

'Sensation without perception' – the failure to recognize familiar objects, although visual, tactile (touch) and auditory systems are unimpaired.

Visual agnosia is loss of visual recognition; other sensory systems can be unaffected: cup, wife or Christmas tree, for example, are not remembered by sight, but may be identifiable by touch, sound or smell. Benton (1979) groups the visual agnosias into:

- Visuoperceptive
    visual object agnosia
    defective visual analysis and synthesis

impaired facial recognition which can manifest as 'prosopagnosia' (of familiar faces) and/or defective discrimination of unfamiliar faces

- Visuospatial
  defective localization of points in space
  defective judgement of direction and distance
  defective topographical orientation
  unilateral neglect.
- Visuoconstructive
  defective assembling performance
  defective graphomotor performance (writing).

Tactile agnosia is also known as 'astereognosis'; not recognizing objects by touch even when sensation is unaltered. This is one of the cognitive tests done routinely by doctors at a first consultation in conjunction with sensory and reflex testing, usually by placing a bunch of keys into the subject's hand whilst their eyes are closed and requesting identification.

Auditory agnosia is not recognizing sounds although hearing is normal.

ANOSODIAPHORIA/EUPHORIA

An abnormal lack of concern about the situation, such as the implications of having had a stroke. This and the next problem are seen mostly in Strokes whose lesion is in the non-dominant hemisphere (usually with L hemiplegia).

Strokes with this impairment in perceptual processing, together with the next more distressing problem, often get labelled as 'unrealistic'. Anosodiaphorics are – and it is unrealistic to expect them to be anything else.

ANOSOGNOSIA

Failure to recognize or understand one's own disability and therefore an inability to relate to it or to remember strategies for dealing with it.

This, like the previous problem, is found in non-dominant hemisphere lesions and can take the form of a personal denial of one or both limbs on the affected side of the body and/or a total inability to comprehend the nature of the stroke state itself, although fully aware of the accompanying handicaps. The first creates confusion for carers; the second can generate tremendous frustration and anxiety for the individual (particularly if they have been good at problem-solving pre-stroke).

This does not respond to reassurance or explanation as the ability to recognize and understand the problems encountered depends on the ability to recognize and understand the disability – it is self-perpetuating.

Anosognosics can appear manipulative – complaining of a lack of treatment or conflicting advice (because rehabilitation for overcoming disabilities which they are unable to recognize is of course not recognized or remembered either). This frequently disturbs working relationships, unless team communication is exemplary (teamwork is examined in Chapter 9). They can also be labelled 'unrealistic' – but anosognosics are desperately attempting to re-establish their parameters.

The solution to the anxiety is to give full explanations and brief reminders as necessary, and to divert attention to something else as discreetly as possible. For rehabilitation purposes a similar programme to that for some dyspraxias using sensory 'prompting' is usually the most helpful (Chapter 10).

APHASIA

Inability to express oneself through speech (expressive dysphasia) or to comprehend the spoken word (receptive dysphasia). These problems frequently extend to written language and to gestures and symbols as well. It is therefore not always useful to hand out picture charts of functional items or activities until a speech therapist has assessed whether it is appropriate. A lesion in the language processing area, which is closely linked with the dominant hemisphere, is usually associated with a R hemiplegia in right-handed people – however aphasia can occur in left-handed people with a L hemiplegia. These problems will be explored further in section 7.5.

APRAXIA/DYSPRAXIA

Movement without perception – the inability to perform certain purposeful movements even though motor power, sensation and intellect may be unimpaired. This is frequently associated with dominant hemisphere lesions, which means this problem is often concealed and/or complicated by aphasia. It is one of the most disabling handicaps in terms of recovery because it affects all the activities of daily living (section 7.3).

DYSLEXIA

'Word blindness' – difficulty in reading, spelling and writing words, despite the ability to see and recognize letters. When it occurs after a stroke or other forms of brain damage, in a person whose reading ability was previously normal, it is called 'acquired dyslexia'.

KINETIC MUTISM

Most often seen in Alzheimer's disease sufferers as a result of the involvement of the dominant pre-frontal cortex, it presents as a physical unresponsiveness to any stimulation – neither voluntary nor automatic movements can be elicited or prompted – although occasional normal responses can sometimes be unexpectedly self-initiated.

LACK OF MOTIVATION

Seldom so simple. Cognitive impairments, secondary pathologies and boredom and fatigue contribute to misunderstanding. This is explored further in Chapter 10.

PERSEVERATION

The persistence or repetition of the same response after the causative stimulus has ceased or in response to a group of different stimuli – it can be one or more words or movements. Discreetly interrupt and introduce the next (anticipated) word, phrase or movement before the repetition becomes self-perpetuating.

UNILATERAL NEGLECT

Ignoring one half of personal near and/or far space. It is particularly associated with lesions in the non-dominant hemisphere so it is often a feature with L hemiplegia. It has nothing to do with hemianopia! Nor with dyspraxia, though it causes confusion with most functional activities.

TO SUMMARIZE

A stroke can result in one or many of these cognitive deficits – and with variable degrees of severity. For many people these impairments are the major obstacles preventing their return to independence and quality of life. Physical disabilities, because they are visible, demand attention, but the invisible ones are often more significant, and a person's failure to adapt or improve in terms of physical ability is frequently misunderstood to be deliberate choice or lack of motivation. Imagine the misery such a label can inflict on someone who is genuinely but helplessly struggling to cooperate.

There are many more cognitive deficits of unknown origin which affect the capacity and speed of the CNS to process information: slowness, sometimes excessive, in responding to exogenous sensory stimulation, to shift from one set of data to another, to organize the units of information and also in the analysis and synthesis of information.

Casebook example

> One Stroke missed several meals although she had made a good
> physical recovery. Escorted to sit in the dayroom after breakfast she
> then stayed there, ignoring requests to join the others for lunch in
> the dining area. Asked if she was hungry she answered 'Yes', but
> stayed where she was. Not lazy, nor unmotivated – merely unable to
> translate the wish into the deed, need into physical action.

Strokes with these executive or 'planning' problems may be unable to
discriminate between essential and non-essential information and can
have difficulty in planning ahead or in foreseeing the implications and
consequences of any action.

7.3 APRAXIA/DYSPRAXIA

This is a disturbance in the programming and execution of volitional,
skilled and purposeful movements in the presence of normal reflexes,
power, tone, coordination and sensation. It is **not** caused by visual, auditory, language, attentional or intellectual impairment, nor by weakness,
abnormality of muscle tone or posture, de-afferation (lack of sensation)
or abnormal movement patterns, poor comprehension or unco-operative
behaviour! (although some or all of these may also be affected by the
stroke).

In 1960 De Ajuriaguerra, Hecaen and Angelergues found constructional dyspraxia in over 60% of their R hemisphere-damaged group, and
in 1966 DeRenzi, Pieczuro and Vignolo discovered 80% of their dys-
phasics to be also dyspraxic (dysphasia is associated with L hemisphere
damage). De Renzi, Motti and Nichelli (1980) identified a dyspraxia in
50% of unpreselected L hemisphere-damaged patients.

As in so many areas of knowledge the terminology is variable, but the
two most frequently encountered dyspraxias, which affect movement
bilaterally, are commonly identified as 'ideomotor' and 'ideational'.

IDEOMOTOR DYSPRAXIA

This is a 'constructional' disorder: impairment in the selection of the
components of a functional movement ('response selection' in Mulder's
model). People with this dyspraxia will often say, 'I know what you are
asking me to do' (e.g. 'put on your shoes'), 'but I don't seem to be able to
do it'. They are not being stupid, they are truly unable to. They are
dyspraxic.

**The performance of even simple motor tasks to command is impos-
sible,** unrelated to any co-existent receptive dysphasia. This inability
extends to the use of gestures – with obvious implications for the learn-

ing of gestural communication systems. However, **automatic movement responses are unimpaired** – therefore ideomotor dyspraxics can function 'on automatic' in everyday situations provided they get the correct environmental clues – apart from some non-fluency of movement seen as a residual clumsiness or awkwardness.

Rehabilitation is based on sub-cortical prompting and teaching auto-initiatives. Problems only arise when the automatic performance is distracted.

Casebook example

'David' regained competent use of his L arm and leg, but movement remained slightly awkward because of the ideomotor dyspraxia. He responded so well to the definitive rehabilitation programme (see Chapter 10) that he was discharged home to continue caring for his wife (she was in the early stage of Alzheimer's disease), and coped fine 'on automatic' using his awareness of auto-initiative strategies when necessary. However, several weeks after his return home, the stroke unit received a call from an irate ambulance driver who had called to collect David for a routine outpatient appointment and found him stranded at the top of the staircase totally unable to proceed downstairs: his wife had interrupted the 'automatic' locomotion to tell him something unrelated to the task on hand. The driver had to put in an emergency call for more ambulance personnel who finally carried Dave bodily downstairs struggling all the way as he tried to explain the simplicity of prompting as an alternative.

Alert ambulance personnel to the possible cognitive problems where appropriate.

IDEATIONAL DYSPRAXIA

This is a 'conceptual' disorder: the inability to carry out purposeful complex sequential acts either to command **or** automatically – a disorder in the 'serial ordering' component of programming in Mulder's model. The stages of the movements and procedures are present, but cannot be put together in the correct order.

For instance: making a cup of tea, for most people, involves taking the lid off the kettle, taking the kettle to the tap, turning on the tap, angling the kettle under the stream of water until it is sufficiently filled, turning off the tap, lifting the kettle clear, replacing the lid, replacing the kettle on the work-surface, plugging the electric cable into the kettle, switching it on at the wall power point, lifting the lid off the teapot, fetching the teacaddy and opening it, spooning out the tealeaves (OK, teabags for some) and into the teapot, switching off the boiling kettle at the wall point, unplugging it, bringing the kettle carefully to the teapot, pouring the contents in, replacing the kettle on the worktop, the teapot lid on the teapot…and then the business of the cup, saucer, spoon, sugar, milk…All complex sequential acts which ideational dyspraxics are quite unable to do, divorcing them from almost all the activities of independent daily life.

There are far too many intricate and hugely disabling apraxias to cover adequately here, but thankfully only a minority (relatively speaking) of Strokes face these afflictions. If you come across someone who displays any of these difficulties quickly refer them to a clinical neuropsychologist, or an occupational therapist specializing in neurological rehabilitation. Cognitive neuropsychology studies the effects that brain injury in humans can have on the cognitive skills, and researches therapeutic strategies.

7.4 UNILATERAL NEGLECT

Clients who may not have elemental sensory or motor defects, but who fail to respond, report or orient to stimuli presented to the side contralateral to the cerebral lesion, have unilateral neglect. This is **not** a visual field detect. It is mostly associated with non-dominant hemisphere lesions (usually L hemiplegia), and affects all activities, for example:

- leaving the S side undressed;
- reading and writing without being aware of the left (S) side of the page (Figure 7.1);
- drawing and even copying drawings leaving areas on the left side of each item in the drawing incomplete or impoverished (Figure 7.2);
- ignoring people or conversation coming from their left;
- knocking into things on their left as they move around;
- being unaware of food or drinks presented or placed to the S side;
- eating only the food on the right side of the plate.

The degree of this impoverishment in representational space (Figure 7.2) often reflects the area of neglect in personal space – the missing bits in drawings correlate with the same areas of unawareness of own-body geography: left hand, or whole arm, part of leg, bits of face, etc. – most noticeable in dressing, putting on make-up, shaving and bruises!

Three of the many theories that are put forward to account for these phenomena are discussed here:

- defective sensory input or defective interpretation of sensory input;
- a disorder of representational schema (the 'inner map' of space);
- impaired attentional or orienting systems.

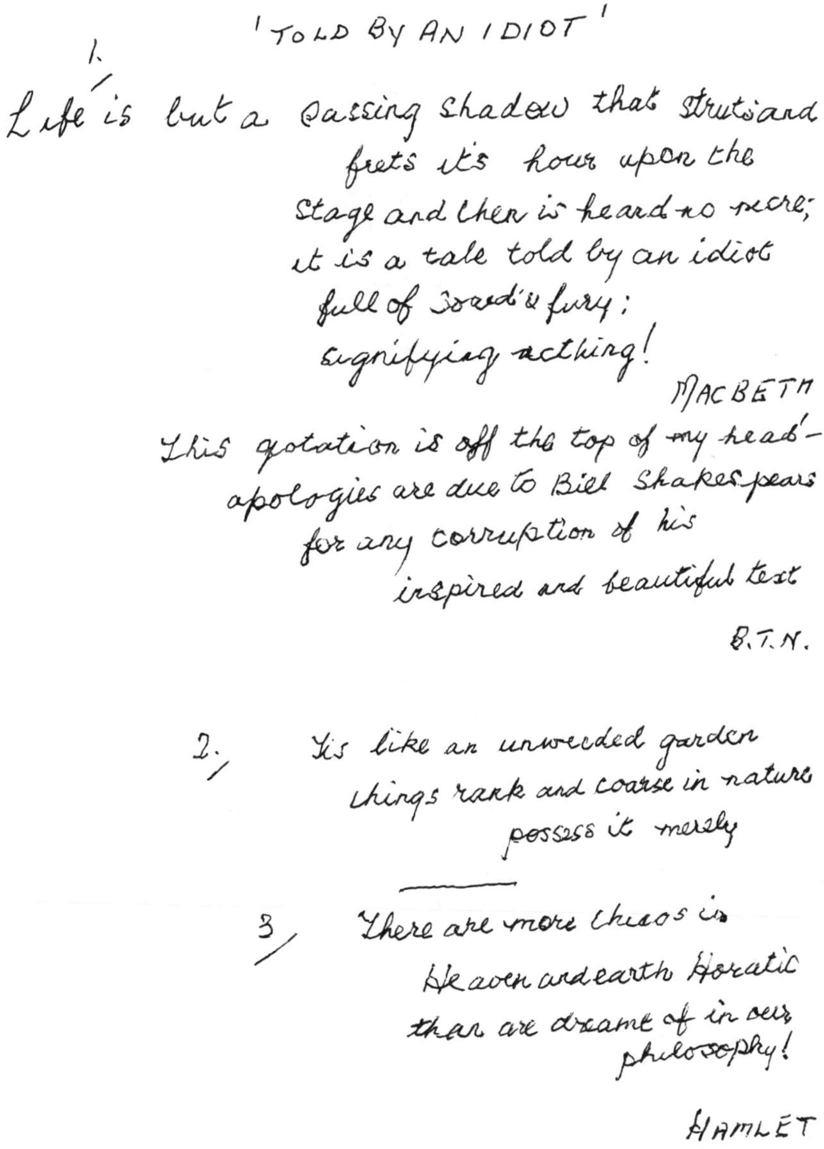

'TOLD BY AN IDIOT'

1.

Life is but a passing shadow that struts and
frets it's hour upon the
stage and then is heard no more;
it is a tale told by an idiot
full of sound's fury:
signifying nothing!

MACBETH

This qotation is off the top of my head—
apologies are due to Bill Shakespeare
for any corruption of his
inspired and beautiful text

B.T.N.

2.
Tis like an unweeded garden
things rank and coarse in nature
possess it merely

3.
There are more chaos in
Heaven and earth Horatio
than are dreamt of in our
philosophy!

HAMLET

Figure 7.1 Unilateral neglect, shown in writing. The title and choice of subject matter indicate the real distress felt by the writer about his post-stroke problems.

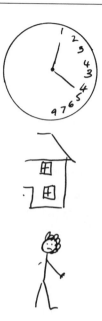

Figure 7.2 Unilateral neglect in drawing and copying.

SENSORY DISTURBANCE

This is certainly not a visual field defect: hemianopia can result from lesions in either hemisphere (you can have a Right or a Left hemianopia), whereas unilateral neglect is most severe in lesions affecting the dominant cerebral hemisphere only.

Sensory defects are not present in many cases of unilateral neglect and, although there are often instances of disturbed interpretation elicited in simultaneous and double simultaneous and two-point sensory stimulation tests, these too are not always present.

DISORDER IN REPRESENTATIONAL SCHEMA

Here the mental (not the actual visible) imagery neglects one side of space. Bisiach and Luzzatti (1978) conducted the following study, which illustrates this very effectively.

In the city of Milan there is an open square, a piazza of great beauty and cultural significance which the local residents are extremely proud of and use as a natural centre both for shopping and promenading. It is the famous Piazza del Duomo, with the great Cathedral at one end and an imposing statue of Victor Emanuel II on his horse at the other. Groups of stroke-afflicted Milanese with known problems of unilateral neglect were taken into a quiet room (one at a time) and, with no visual reminder available, invited to imagine themselves standing with their back to the statue and facing across the concourse to the Cathedral. They were then asked to name in sequence all the buildings around the Piazza that they could 'see' in their mind's eye, so to speak. The answers were remarkably consistent – they listed those to the right of the Cathedral but omitted most of those on the left-hand side. They were then told to imagine themselves standing at the other end of the Piazza with their back to the Cathedral and facing towards the statue, and again asked to name the buildings in sequence. Again, all those to the right of the Piazza were listed – which were, of course, those omitted the first time – but not those on the left (which they had 'seen' and listed the first time). When the missing buildings were described to them they were able to name them – they did know them all, but were quite unable to 'visualize' the left side of space in their mental imagery.

ATTENTIONAL THEORY OF NEGLECT

This can be demonstrated in various forms one of which is as a hemispatial akinesia – an inability to initiate an action in or towards the contralateral hemisphere. It is suggested that the reticular bounceback of sensory input fails to alert the damaged hemisphere.

Springer and Deutsch (1989) and Kosslyn (1988) found in electroencephalogram (EEG) studies that EEG activity increases in the R hemisphere during spatial tasks, indicating that this hemisphere could be responsible for global visualization or attentional schema. Certain lesions in the R hemisphere would then demonstrate unilateral neglect.

When asked to bisect a horizontal line, people with unilateral neglect tend to choose a point to the right of true midpoint. Sometimes this tendency can be reduced if a cue such as a coloured mark or flashing light is presented at the left-hand end of the horizontal line.

Riddoch and Humphreys (1983) showed that cueing was only really effective if the person was made to report the cue each time, suggesting that neglect may be a more serious impairment of automatic rather than of deliberate attentional orienting. This gives some clue to the development of strategies for rehabilitation.

What happens to all this 'neglected' information? Reasoning can be sound and there is possibly a covert awareness, but excuses and denial come naturally with this problem. In one study which involved copying a simple line drawing of a house with smoke and flames issuing from a left-hand upper window, the participant successfully drew the house but omitted the window and the fire. When his attention was drawn to it, and he was asked why he hadn't included it in his drawing, he at first denied that it was there and then declared that he chose to live in a non-burning house.

People with these severe forms of unilateral neglect, like the dyspraxics, seldom achieve true independence. They are sometimes quite unaware of their plight, and rehabilitation to independent functional status depends largely on rebuilding the lost spatial awareness – and reinforcing awareness of their problem.

Casebook example

> 'Harry' had made a good physical recovery, but with the hidden deficit of unilateral neglect to his left of which he remained persistently unaware and continued to deny. His overriding desire was to return to driving a car and all the explanations and counselling regarding the obvious (to his therapists) impracticability failed to convince him. In order to get his driving licence reissued he required a doctor's certificate declaring his ability, and his family physician, having checked the recovery in the hemiplegic arm and leg and impressed by Harry's obviously normal intellect in conversation, enthusiastically agreed. It was when the formal driving licence application form arrived that he began to have doubts. His patient presented himself in the consulting room waving the document and complaining bitterly that it was stupid, unintelligible and a disgraceful example of mindless bureaucracy. Doctor, patient and the offending form duly arrived in the stroke unit seeking guidance. Read aloud word by word any page of any book or document that has a wide strip of the writing obliterated on the left-hand side, and the dilemma becomes obvious: what remains does not make sense. This incident finally persuaded the would-be driver that he did have difficulties and highlighted – to the doctor – the perceptual difficulties that can result from a stroke.

Specialized Driving Assessment Centres are recommended for Strokes who wish to return to driving; they will also advise on appropriate modifications.

7.5 LANGUAGE

(**Dysarthria** results from somatic and sensory system impairment affecting articulation, phonation and resonance, which presents difficulties in the lowest level of speech – the production of speech sounds. The command of language remains intact, but speech is slowed and slurred; volume is diminished and pitch or intonation can be distorted. These have been described in the previous chapter on abnormal function: they are not the result of cognitive deficits.)

DYSPRAXIA

Dyspraxia of speech, as with dyspraxias of movement outlined in section 7.3, is specifically a cognitive dysfunction affecting coordination and sequencing of the articulatory musculature. It presents as a problem in language production and can occur without dysarthria and with word-finding skills remaining unimpaired. Accurate positioning of the articulators for the formation of recognisable speech, as well as the correct sequencing of responses, can be affected.

The effortful and repetitive attempts to produce sounds correctly, made by Strokes with articulatory dyspraxia, disrupt both vowels and consonants and affect the timing and coordination of voice onset time. It is most obvious as an initiation difficulty, and is displayed as false starts and restarts as the subject visibly 'gropes' for lip and tongue organization. Evidence is mounting that many of the speech errors and nonspeech 'gropings' can be explained by models of motor control and learning (Wertz et al., 1984).

DYSPHASIA

This is a disturbance of language at the second and third levels, resulting from damage to the language processing area which includes expressive and receptive language in both spoken and written forms. The problems, like language, are infinitely complex and this is a brief outline only.

Expressive problems present as an inability to:

- retrieve words to express;
- retrieve appropriate words;
- sequence words in their correct order;

i.e. difficulties in word finding, word selection and grammatical construction.

Sometimes prefixes and suffixes are omitted or used indiscriminately – a diabetic Stroke was quizzed on diet by an anxious Consultant prior to discharge home: 'How can you manage a nourishing meal on the days the meals-on-wheels service doesn't deliver?' The effortful reply included a thoroughly satisfactory answer '...eggles... bananakins ...'

The lexicon can be selectively blitzed by the lesion, so that certain groups of words seem to remain inaccessible even when some recovery of language has been achieved. These problems have titles of their own within the generic label of dysphasia, like 'anomia': the inability to retrieve the names of persons or objects. This problem is often compensated for by circumlocution, paraphrasing around the missing word.

Casebook examples

- Another Stroke about to be discharged from hospital to live alone was interrogated by the same anxious Consultant: 'We have to arrange community services for you – where do you live?' An agonized silence ended in triumph: 'That arty farty place' – instantly identified as a nearby very trendy small town.

- The wife of one Stroke was really dismayed by his continuing failure to produce her name in any context. After 25 good years of marriage her husband could only refer to her as 'she', or, when pressed, as 'you know, the woman I married'. The same Stroke recovered much of his working language – except for names – over a period of about two years and, unable to return to farming because of his severe residual physical handicaps, he both achieved and received much confidence as a prison visitor counselling long-term prisoners. His own frustrations and loss of physical 'freedom' gave him an extra empathy and gained him great respect. He described the struggle to locate and correctly select words as, 'Crawling down a narrow tunnel towards a word. If, when I get to it, it's the wrong word, then I have to back out and head down the next tunnel. Sometimes I am still holding the wrong word and have to struggle to get rid of it – when I find the correct word I have to drag it out of the tunnel and hold on to it while I surface and try to put it into place.'

As with re-programmed movement, nothing is as easy after a stroke as it was before.

Jargon results from the inability to recognize and/or select approriate words. It is fluent speech without meaning – to the hearer that is – the speaker is usually satisfied that the selection of words perfectly conveys the message and is confused only by the recipient's lack of comprehension. Sometimes an occasional word in amongst the rest is correct or close and the gist of the conversation can be understood or guessed at.

Perseveration is the repetition of a word or a phrase, which precludes ongoing meaningful conversation.

Ongoing loss or **disturbance** of speech is often considered to be a worse handicap than the physical disabilities, especially by families and friends who sometimes associate it with a total loss of 'mental' faculties. However, there are many other methods of communication which, although not as satisfactory as the previous 'normal', will supplement the gaps for conveying purposeful messages and enable participation in social conversation.

The simplest and most effective of these are the gestural systems: Amer-Ind for instance provides a basically familiar and easily learned alternative (some of the Amer-Ind vocabulary is illustrated in Chapter 14). Some Strokes and families develop their own gestural language from familiar and recognized habitual signalling.

Gesture, body language, facial expressions, etc. are naturally used in everyday situations, and also serve to stimulate returning – or the re-learning of – language skills. The Stroke who described his word-finding in such vivid terms also used the entire range of physical expression, and could relate anecdotes and funny stories with consummate skill (and waiting for the punchline added to its punch).

Abstract thought is difficult to portray and it is often this loss of verbal individuality that creates such frustration.

Receptive problems include the inability to decode words, to work out their meaning. This is an even greater disability in terms of social isolation and aggravation, but here again the use of body language, gestural communication, etc. by everyone else can help to bridge the language barrier.

In trying to explain the situation to Strokes and their relatives/friends, the dysphasia of stroke can be likened to finding oneself – without warning – in another country where the native language is not known. The traveller is still the same intelligent, educated individual, but unable to converse in or comprehend the local tongue. Some words may be the same, or recalled from previous foreign language forays; used in conjunction with gestures and mime this can be adequate in many situations for both expressing oneself and comprehending others. Sometimes quite a vocabulary can be learned or recalled, but occasionally the speech sounds remain unreproducible and unrecognized or meaningless to the local population.

Some gestures too have different interpretations in other countries. In a series of multidisciplinary workshops (on the management of stroke) in Malta, the basic gestural Amer-Ind vocabulary was greeted with such delight that the expanded and more socially conversational Amer-Ind was added to the programme. Suddenly the participants appeared to lose concentration and the session broke up in disarray. Afterwards it was explained to us that the gestures for 'Good Morning' (accompanied by a wide smile) in Amer-Ind signify 'Homosexual is Good' in Malta.

Certain spoken words can be utilized for multiple meanings when used in conjunction with gesture, e.g. 'food' can indicate anything edible, or a specific item or dish, or mealtimes, the preparation of food, ingredients or being hungry. I lived and worked for a while in Arabic countries and was never able to produce the glottal speech sounds necessary to speak any of the arabic languages – so communication was primarily gestural with nouns and verbs (usually mispronounced) without glottal sounds or grammatical construction. It worked surprisingly well and I was never labelled 'disabled' or made to feel inadequate. People laughed with me as I groped for words, but never at me: they understood my difficulties, giving clues and prompting when I got stuck and complementing their conversation with vivid mime: no problem (thumbs up, wide smile).

Rehabilitation of dysphasia requires the guidance of an expert speech and language therapist and the inclusion of Stroke partners and all carers in the process. Learning a basic gestural communication system and using it with appropriate embellishments in all situations will help everyone to communicate (including other Strokes and any visitors) and also encourage the language-impaired Strokes to participate in – and not to feel excluded from – all social and sociable activities.

Go through what is comprehensible and you conclude that only the incomprehensible gives any light.

(Saul Bellow)

REFERENCES

Benton, A.L. (1979) Visuoperceptive, visuospatial and visuoconstructive disorders, in *Clinical Neuropsychology*, (eds K.M. Heilman and E. Valenstein), Oxford University Press, New York.

Bisiach, E. and Luzzatti, C. (1978) Unilateral neglect of representational space. *Cortex*, **14**, 129–33.

De Renzi, E., Motti, F. and Nichelli, P. (1980) Imitating gestures: a quantitative approach to ideomotor dyspraxia. *Archives of Neurology*, **37**, 6–10.

Kosslyn, S.M. (1988) Aspects of a cognitive neuroscience of mental imagery. *Science*, **240**, 1621–6.

Riddoch, M.J. and Humphreys, G.W. (1983) The effect of cueing on unilateral neglect. *Neuropsychologia*, **21**, 589–99.

Springer, S.P. and Deutsch, G. (1989) *Left Brain, Right Brain*, 3rd edn, Freeman, San Francisco.

Wertz, R., La Pointe, L. and Rosenbek, J. (1984) *Apraxia of Speech in Adults*, Grune & Stratton, New York.

Lame dogmas

8

Dogma does not mean absence of thought, but the end of thought.
(G.K. Chesterton)

Stroke and stroke rehabilitation, like religion, has been bedevilled by conflicting ideologies and fleeting fads. Even now, despite the advancing Age of Enlightenment, bad habits and adverse adages are rife. With growing awareness of the plasticity of the human neuromuscular system, the old axioms need to be rewritten, re-evaluated or completely thrown out before even more Strokes are moulded into the twisted patterns of traditional disablement or transferred to 'Homes for the Bewildered' (as they are labelled by Dame Edna Everage).

Although much of the following inappropriate practice has been eradicated, some or all of it is still earnestly practised. In fact, several are appropriate – but only in certain circumstances; this aspect is emphasized where relevant.

Each 'lame dogma' identified in this chapter will be described and then analysed, with exceptions noted in italics. The list is undoubtedly incomplete and, as understanding of CNS control increases, many more of the existing techniques and approaches may have to be jettisoned – so continue to question these and prepare to be ruthless: **outdated doctrines can disable**.

1 'SQUEEZE A (?TENNIS) BALL'

Terrible in its simplicity, this little piece of advice is still handed out (sometimes with the ball) by misguided professionals and well-intentioned friends as an exercise to restore hand movement.

What it actually does is to stimulate and reinforce the primitive grasp reflex, leading, very quickly indeed, to a clawed, unremediable hand and increasing spasticity of the whole upper limb. Grip alone is useless without the ability to open the hand, first to grasp objects and then to release them.

Exception

*Moulding the hand round a ball or cone, and holding it (but **not** squeezing it), can sometimes benefit the minority of Strokes who develop the 'shoulder-hand' syndrome with flaccidity of muscle tone and eventual rigidity or hyperextension of the metacarpo-phalangeal (knuckle) joints. This needs to be expertly identified first. If the presence of an object in the hand stimulates the grasp reflex (the tip of the thumb is often clawing anyway), then don't do it.*

2 FORCED PASSIVE STRETCHING STRAIGHTENS OUT SPASTICITY

Tempting, but utterly traumatic.

'Spastic' musculature lacks reciprocal innervation, movement produces uninhibited contraction: forced lengthening starts by stimulating increased contraction (remember the 'stretch reflex'?) and ends by rupturing muscle fibres.

Pulling on curled fingers can hyper-extend the metacarpo-phalangeal joints – so does allowing the Stroke to forcibly flatten the fingers (by leaning on them) with the wrist flexed. Full dorsiflexion (up) of the wrist with full extension of the fingers is unnatural (try it). Subsequent pain increases the reflex response; it goes from bad to worse.

If full-range finger movements are wanted, start with the wrist in full plantarflexion (down), and don't stress any joints. Muscles work over joints: stretching spastic muscle, therefore, also stresses unprotected joints and damages the ligaments and connective tissue girdling.

Casebook example

An enthusiastic consultant physician became impatient with a Stroke who presented with severe flexor hyper-reflexia, having been chair-bound for several weeks prior to admission to a stroke unit. Having tried to straighten the S leg (to test muscle strength! See 4) and failed, the doctor lifted the S leg on to a footstool (with the knee still at a right-angle, reflexia now reinforced by the increased flexion at the hip) and, pre-empting intervention from onlookers, with both hands and full bodyweight, forcibly slammed the S knee down into near-extension. Within 30 minutes the joint had blown up to nightmare proportions and the orthopaedic team had to be rushed in. For four weeks active rehabilitation for the Stroke was hampered while the S knee was subjected to serial drainage of blood and fluid, became infected, was irreversibly damaged, and full range of movement and normal gait were permanently impaired, although the original hyper-reflexia responded to skilled therapy and recovery from the stroke itself was good.

3 'LACK OF MOTIVATION'

Generally means, 'reduced to despair' unless there is a lesion which has damaged the processing of incoming signals, in which case both verbal and physical prompting may always be needed.

Screen for: anxiety, depression, cognitive dysfunction including dyspraxias, language comprehension and object recognition, general health (urine retention, constipation/faecal impaction, urinary/chest infections, cardiac function – a client on one stroke unit appeared to come to a complete standstill until fitted with a cardiac pacemaker), Parkinsonian traits, tactless or patronizing intervention (many Strokes and their families are told within a couple of weeks after the event that, 'He/she will never walk/talk again', etc.) and sheer boredom.

Rehabilitation does not have to be dull, humourless, painful, ineffectual, apparently weird or motiveless (do explain to people what sitting on a wobble-board – or standing up being randomly shoved in the back by a therapist – has to do with learning how to walk again).

Remember the implications for neurological rehabilitation in recent findings: that the practising of non-functional exercises cannot assist in the performance of functional activity.

Introduce familiar task- and context-specific activities, different environments, and intersperse serious activities with easily-accomplished and occasionally frivolous tasks.

4 TESTING MUSCLE STRENGTH

The usual tests applied by persons who think that the motor disabilities of stroke are the result of muscle-weakness, and that strength of response indicates degree of impairment and progress.

- 'Squeeze my hand', which equates with squeezing a tennis ball,
- 'Bend your arm' against the resistance of tester's hand on the Stroke's wrist and
- 'Straighten your leg', against the resistance of tester's hand on the S shin,

stimulate all the associated primitive reflex patterns in trunk and limbs and enhance abnormalities in muscle tone.

The resulting actions are the product of pathological neuromuscular changes, such as spastic reflexia, and as such are no indicators of normal muscle strength or weakness, only of already predictable abnormality.

Strength is only one of the complex components of normal movement, and usually the least significant following any CNS trauma, so the attempt to test it in isolation is at best unhelpful and at worst damaging to recovery (as well as daft).

5 'MONKEY-POLES' AND COTSIDES ARE NECESSARY

Heaving oneself around the bed using an over-bed pulley (in the N hand) produces almost ineradicable gross extensor reflexia, and only succeeds in beaching the body across the bed like a stranded whale. Attempting to use the S hand too will reinforce the grasp reflex and probably irretrievably traumatize the vulnerable glenohumeral joint.

Cotsides encourage pulling (same result, disabling reflexia). Placing the bed so that the S side is to the wall (mistakenly seen as the alternative safety precaution) confirms hyperactivity to the N side and reinforces unilateral neglect.

Exception

A cotside may be required in certain cases (see Chapter 10).

6 CURRENT ABILITY DETERMINES FUTURE COMPETENCE

Not likely! Predictive assessment based on ongoing assessment gives some idea, but if enlightened rehabilitation is started early enough – and with ongoing encouragement – the Stroke will continue to progress indefinitely. The provision of aids and equipment needs constant review to enable this, particularly in the home environment.

Exception

Certain cognitive impairments can seriously affect the recovery of functional independence (Chapter 10 includes a simple checklist towards predicting outcome).

7 GOOD RECOVERY FROM A STROKE IS DUE TO HARD WORK AND GOOD MOTIVATION – AND VICE VERSA

A common enough pronouncement (usually by doctors trying to instil hope into a drooping patient), but sadly it is not entirely accurate.

It is often applied (retrospectively) to the fortunate few who have had a relatively slight stroke with apparently few residual disabilities. These are frequently held up as a good example to others – which is desperately unfair to the Stroke who has worked hard to overcome or reduce more severe disablement resulting from larger or more disadvantageous lesions and is still left with considerable handicaps.

The converse (poor recovery is due to insufficient hard work and/or poor motivation) is entirely inaccurate – see the preceding statement – or the Stroke may have worked hard and enthusiastically, but the rehabilitation programmes may not have been good enough.

Exception

Absolutely true when applied to the rehabilitation team, though.

8 'WORK – OR TRY – HARDER'

Those that can, do; those that don't, usually can't. (Those that won't probably won't; some people are naturally contrary.)

- physical effort produces and reinforces hyper-reflexia; increasing effort leads to spasticity. Performance doesn't improve, it deteriorates. Try harder to get worse?
- stamina is affected by stroke. In addition to possible partial denervation of muscle, the concentration required to reproduce consciously the formerly automatic postural background which enables compliance with given tasks, let alone that required for the task itself, is immense – any reserves of energy are quickly depleted.
- many strokes with cognitive impairment are genuinely unable to initiate activity without appropriate clueing and prompting. Left to themselves they are helpless through no fault of their own and nagging will only compound their misery.

Exceptions

Natural or clinical depression can present as lethargy: reassurance that endeavour will be assisted – and rewarded – by improvement may help to break the spell.

There will always be individuals who are naturally content to let the world go by: urging and nagging probably won't change the situation or benefit the Stroke, but carers may feel better for it.

9 GOAL-SETTING WITH THE STROKE

This depends absolutely upon realistic assessment of the situation and the relationship between the Stroke and the goal-setter.

- Unrealistic targets are usually unreachable and create depression in all concerned.
- Time-related targets can cause anxiety and excessive effort (which precipitates hyper-reflexia and fatigue) and the keen practising of activities unsupervised, which may result in the development of unnecessary or abnormal compensatory movement patterns.

Exception

Realistic planning is the important factor. Timing may be a necessary factor in clinical audit (but try not to inflict it on the Stroke).

10 GOING BACK TO BED FOR A REST IS 'GIVING IN'

It is not, it is recuperative and rehabilitative (Chapter 10). The alternative – dozing in a slumped position in a chair – is detrimental and reinforces abnormal postures.

Exception

Staying *in bed might be ...*

11 SITTING CORRECTLY PREVENTS SPASTICITY

Not for long. Remaining in one position for any length of time actually invokes underlying reflexive patterning.

Sitting with the S leg flexed at the hip and with the knee and foot in dorsiflexion on the floor for most of the day will enhance the flexor pattern and the PSR (Positive Supporting Reaction) making future walking almost impossible.

The Stroke featured in lame dogma 2 had been 'correctly' positioned like this during the day every day for several weeks, with the result that the hyper-reflexia was so strong that when nurses tried to get him to stand up from sitting (in a chair or on the edge of the bed), the poor man doubled up into a ball (trunk flexors snapping into action on feeling the sudden stretch) and toppled forwards on to the floor, head first. When picked up he hung between them in full flexion again. Strategies to overcome this are described in Chapter 10.

Similarly, if the S leg is propped up on a footstool for long enough (usually joined by the N leg for comfort) this promotes the full extensor patterning.

The same applies to sustained S arm and hand positions.

Exception

*Reflex-inhibiting positions are important to prevent the development of latent spasticity, but **only** if they are altered frequently enough – so alert everyone! Let the Stroke spend an hour or so with feet positioned on floor, another hour with feet on footstool, and plenty of natural breaks (which involve standing) for toileting, transfers, mealtimes, etc. This is especially important for Strokes who already display hyper-reflexic tendencies. It also reintroduces natural dynamics, prevents pressure sores, increases activity and reduces boredom.*

12 STRIP THE STROKE FOR PHYSICAL THERAPY

The struggle to undress and get into little shorts usually gets the Stroke thoroughly screwed up so that the ensuing treatment session is devoted to smoothing everything out again. This is perhaps satisfying for the therapist, but not very progressive for the Stroke (really useful for demonstrating inhibitory techniques, though).

Elderly Strokes are often embarrassed (near-nakedness in a small consulting room takes courage for some, let alone in a busy and fairly public department – and curtains are no comfort and also isolate the client quite unnecessarily from the rest of the world). Room temperature is usually set for the fully dressed (the therapists) or the active, and any self-consciousness is heightened by personal disability. It takes an experienced and skilled therapist to achieve the total concentration needed from the Stroke to overcome these conditions and gain an increase in ability.

Most rehabilitation can be successfully progressed without watching the skin surface. Hands-on 'feeling' of the muscle response to strategies is much more educational for the therapist (and more socially acceptable and less distracting to the Stroke through thin ordinary clothing).

Exception

Occasional stripping-off for assessment purposes is essential. For demonstrating specific physical blips in performance it is only necessary to expose the relevant areas: shoulders, trunk or feet for instance (the wearing of a singlet under top clothes is helpful.) Of course if the stripping/dressing routine is facilitated as part of the treatment episode, then this makes it all a bit more therapeutic! These procedures are detailed in Chapter 13. Also younger Strokes who are sports-orientated often relish the opportunity to get back into a familiar training role.

13 GET FULL RANGE OF MOVEMENT (ROM) IN THE S SHOULDER

Only causes trauma unless the full normal shoulder-girdle movement is free and under normal muscular control. Pain is not always felt until the damage is done (because of sensory impairment) and then it is usually the result of chronic trauma. The glenohumeral joint is most at risk, but the muscles which sandwich the scapula into place can suffer too (Figure 8.1).

Restricted normal RoM after a stroke will be due to hyper-reflexia of trunk musculature and spastic abnormal patterning – or pain due to already traumatised tissues – or adhesions following repetitive trauma (probably through ignorant handling and/or mistaken attempts to gain full RoM).

Self-assisted movement (the Stroke hauling the S arm into elevation, or forward-reaching, with the N arm) will stimulate trunk extension anyway

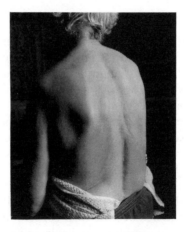

Figure 8.1 Uprooted scapula, from forcing arm movements against spasticity.

(to stabilize the extra weight: try it for yourself) and abnormal hyper-reflexia (because of the effort involved), and can even dislocate a S glenohumeral joint unsupported by normal synergic muscle activity (in addition to traumatizing the connective tissue and ligaments surrounding the joint) just as in the injudicious helper-assisted arm movements.

Moulding or strapping the S hand to a pulley, for hauling up and down with the N hand, is an appalling exercise still used in some places that results in forcible stretching, which causes even more severe trauma to the S shoulder.

Gripping the medial border of the scapula and forcibly assisting this to move inflicts further damage to musculature which is in the contracting mode set by post-stroke trunk hypertonia – even if the muscles themselves are hypotonic (in which case they are subject to damage from overstretching).

How often is full arm elevation necessary in everyday activity anyway? Even hair-brushing is performed with the glenohumeral joint in midline – and many elderly Strokes have acquired limited RoM already. Enquire about previous trauma, compare with the N arm and always relate to predicted need prior to any intervention. Figure 8.1 shows the result of forced passive (euphemistically, 'assisted active') movement in the attempt to gain full RoM of the arm. Treat the cause and the effect.

14 IF IT HURTS IT'S DOING YOU GOOD

If it hurts it is damaging soft-tissue structures, or putting pressure on already damaged joints.

Stroke rehabilitation should **never** be painful – investigate, reassess, analyse, treat the pain and the cause – and amend the activity accordingly.

15 DROPPED SHOULDER ON THE S SIDE IS THE PROBLEM

Not often! The problem is usually that the N shoulder is raised and over-active, creating the illusion of a dropped shoulder on the other (S) side. Ask the Stroke to relax ('drop') the N shoulder, and reassess.

Exception

If the musculature is hypotonic, then a degree of gravitational drop may well be present. It is seldom significant unless other structures are compromised (if it produces undue tension in the nerves of the cervical plexus, for example).

Subluxation is not the same problem, although with hypotonic shoulder musculature the glenohumeral joint is probably subluxed too.

16 THE 'HEMI-CUFF' IS THE SOLUTION

The 'hemi-cuff' support, which straps around the upper part of the S arm and relies on a firm figure-of-eight strap across the nape of the neck under the N shoulder to hold the S glenohumeral joint in place, has been well proven to be totally ineffective for this purpose.

   The correct application confuses most carers, and the taut tension required to approximate the S joint causes painful pressure in the N axilla. Even a slight wriggle to ease the discomfort necessitates re-positioning of the angle of pull up into the S glenohumeral joint, every time, by an experienced helper (the Stroke cannot achieve this because the wriggle factor is involved in self-application: a 'Catch-22' situation). More effective solutions are to be found in Chapter 10.

17 BILATERAL TASKS HASTEN RECOVERY

Not for long. Endless polishing or sanding sessions with the N hand controlling the S arm merely exercises the N arm.

   It can also contribute to malalignment of the glenohumeral joint in a hypotonic limb, and the popular wall-mounted games and activities can traumatize the S shoulder also by the forcible stretching of spastic musculature.

Exception

*Facilitation of **naturally** bilateral activity does hasten recovery (Chapter 10).*

18 PARALLEL BARS ASSIST WALKING

Not merely useless – totally counter-productive.

Stable fixtures for the upper limbs provide fixed external reaction for quadrupedal gait (the floor provides for the lower limbs) and prevents the relearning of dynamic postural control.

Equilibrium reactions are replaced by reinforced dependency on four-point control.

Upper limb pulling, pushing and grabbing replaces normal use of the lower limbs for support and locomotion.

The bars themselves provoke grabbing and pulling which reinforces the spasticity of hyper-reflexive patterning.

A suitable alternative is recommended in Chapter 10.

19 WALKING IS TOP PRIORITY

No, dynamic postural control against gravity is top priority.

Walking, before this is established, creates a sense of insecurity and stimulates all the abnormal reflex patterns, which are then reinforced by the ensuing poor gait.

20 WALKING-SPEED OVER A SET DISTANCE IS IMPORTANT

It may indicate the degree of recovery achieved in relatively slight strokes, but only if no abnormal postures or reflex limb activity can be identified during the walk. To increase speed, the ball of the rear foot needs to 'push-off' to propel the bodyweight forwards. Each step-through with the N leg therefore triggers the PSR in the S limb for the majority of Strokes – so normal gait is immediately destroyed. Challenging the more severely disabled Stroke in this way can undo months of careful rehabilitation, and creates an unnecessary parameter: is fast lop-sided walking more important in everyday life than a slower more normal gait? Uneven gait produces abnormal stresses on all weight-bearing structures too, which precipitate other long-term problems.

Exception

Some studies indicate that timed walking can predict recovery time. Yes, possibly, in that it indicates the validity of motor control systems, but surely this is better assessed (and more revealingly) using other, less disabling, means? Then again no, because it does not demonstrate any factor other than locomotion, which is seldom related to a functional recovery, i.e. of the activities of daily living.

Many elderly Strokes appear to have made an excellently quick recovery if timed walking is an indication; staff in the psychogeriatric day centres, where many of these poor souls end up due to cognitive impairments, spend a lot of time retrieving them from around the countryside.

21 'DROPPED FOOT'

This is only one part of a gross abnormal pattern, not a problem in one isolated component, and should not be treated as such.

Do not issue a rigid orthosis **or** prop up against a footboard in bed – this stimulates the Positive Supporting Reflex (which has probably caused the problem in the first place) and prevents recovery of an acceptably normal or near-normal gait.

Inhibit the gross reflexia, facilitate the normal gross movement and the component part will respond.

22 SPASTICITY HELPS WALKING

Another all-too-frequent misapprehension, usually applied to hypotonic Strokes further handicapped by potential hyper-reflexia (possibly mistaken for normal supporting reactions which **are** required, see Chapter 10).

Eliciting extensor thrust in the S leg includes plantarflexion and inversion of the S foot, and also stimulates the unilateral trunk reactions and upper limb reflexes.

'Crab-like gait is normal after stroke' comes into the same category. It demonstrates uninhibited trunk hyper-reflexia and is abnormal and remediable. Unchecked, it results in worsening disablement, postural insecurity and orthopaedic problems (pathological changes in weight-bearing joints, intervertebral disc distortion with pressure on peripheral nerves, and so on).

If people can 'walk' with spasticity, they can walk even better without it.

23 STEP FORWARD WITH THE STROKE LEG FIRST

And reinforce uninhibited reflexia and the traditional disabilities?

The stereotyped abnormal patterning seen in stroke involves hip flexion, knee extension, foot plantarflexion and inversion on the S side, and also pelvic 'rotation' backwards. Try it: stuck in this position the S leg can only be prodded forwards first. It is tiring. It is not 'walking'.

Always initiate stepping and walking with the N leg – 'best foot forwards' is easy to remember. This breaks up the reflex pattern (extending the S hip) and transfers bodyweight to the standing (S) leg to stimulate the secondary self-inhibitory mechanisms in preparation for the next phase: the follow-through step with the N leg.

24 PEDALLING HELPS MOBILITY

No! It increases spasticity! Whether on a stationary exercise bike or a free-standing set wedged against the wall, pedalling provokes all the stereotyped reflex patterns as the S leg flexes and extends from the hip, and the push down with the ball of the S foot creates havoc.

Even worse, the S foot is sometimes strapped on to the pedal to prevent it shooting off. The trapped plantarflexed and inverted foot of the extended and thrusting leg then forces the pelvis up to throw even more weight on to the N side, reinforcing the problem.

Exception

*Strokes who have regained good functional movement with **no** latent abnormal reflexes can cope with it – but these are rare indeed.*

25 WALKING AIDS/SPLINTS ARE NEVER SUPPLIED BY GOOD THERAPISTS

Good therapists supply whatever is appropriate to facilitate normal locomotion. It is better to walk well with a stick and/or a 'lively' (flexible) splint than badly without one.

Exception

Never supply rigid orthoses and four-legged Zimmer frames. Grasping this frame is necessary for the lift forward between steps, which triggers the primitive grasp reflex – and the lift itself triggers the abnormal reflex patterning in the upper limbs and the trunk. The tendency is to rear backwards snatching the frame to the bosom. This is a walking aid?
A rollator is OK (Chapter 10).

26 USE A HIGH STICK

Encourages raised N shoulder and further side flexion in the S side, reinforcing unilateral trunk hyper-reflexia and the lopsided gait of an apparently shortened S leg.

Exception

Recommended when the Stroke has marked sensory impairment in the lower limb and compensates by leaning and weight-bearing to the N side – or has no need of the support offered by the stick, but requires a little sense of security.

Using a high stick held centrally in both hands in front of the body is a strategy sometimes promoted to re-educate centralized dynamic balance in walking. However, walking with both arms fixed centrally forward is not conducive to normal gait which requires freely-alternating arm swing with trunk rotation, so this manoeuvre is very seldom justifiable.

27 'CONFUSED/INTELLECTUALLY IMPAIRED/DEMENTED'

Unacceptable until properly assessed.

These adjectives are frequently recorded in medical files, and tend to accompany the Stroke into all ongoing formal episodes of care – and are often relayed to the family and/or carers also – affecting attitudes, expectations and options for ongoing rehabilitation.

Investigate the pre-stroke status: if the label refers only to the post-stroke state, then investigate cognitive malfunctioning, which is usually remediable or modifiable given appropriate rehabilitation.

Casebook example

> One Stroke was labelled demented after creating havoc at meal-times – she tipped-up sugar bowls, cups of tea and, although she had recovered reasonably functional movement in her upper limb, appeared to be deliberately choosing not to feed herself. A psychological assessment diagnosed behavioural problems and she became increasingly aggressive. Long-term care in a psychogeriatric unit (at the age of 57) was scheduled, to the obvious grief of her family (two sons with their own families) and many friends. Her complete expressive aphasia further complicated the issue, as did the fact that the therapists found her to be enthusiastic and well-motivated in their own departments.
>
> A joint assessment was finally arranged which began with a cosy cup of coffee in the physiotherapy department. Mrs Davies was discovered to be:
>
> - totally deaf (gestural communication and mime solved this);
> - patchily agnosic, i.e. she couldn't recognize the cup, but when her hands were folded around it and guided to her mouth and drinking was facilitated, Eureka!

A couple of weeks spent re-acquainting her with all the objects she might encounter in daily life and she was the darling of the ward, helping nurses to make beds and other Strokes to keep optimistic. She was soon confident enough to return to living alone in her own home, with a little support from family and friends. Her gratitude was embarrassing to the therapists concerned, who had intervened – almost too late – only because a student nurse knew the family and was herself distressed to see a friend behaving so out of character (teamwork is discussed in Chapter 9).

Communication problems, agnosias and the dyspraxias are the most frequent causes of misunderstanding. Just being misunderstood is enough to dement anyone.

Exception

Pre-stroke confusion/dementia requires historical perspective – and the advice of the professionals previously involved – to achieve rehabilitation from the stroke.

However, always check the origin of pre-stroke confusion: this may be the result of an unrecognized previous minor stroke which itself is remediable...

28 ICING PROMOTES NORMAL MUSCLE TONE

It momentarily modifies spasticity to allow facilitation of hypotonic musculature, but the hypertonia returns and is likely to increase after each application.

Only strategies which promote **auto-inhibitory** responses promote ongoing normalization of muscle tonus.

Plunging a limb, or part of a limb, into ice slush or iced water produces fast vaso-constriction causing an equally fast up-shoot in blood pressure. As the initial stroke in many cases has been the consequence of raised blood pressure, this technique cannot be recommended for general use.

Icing around the mouth and lips or over the left shoulder is thought to affect cardiac function through connections with the autonomic nervous system network and the vagus nerve. Although not proven to be counter-productive, perhaps it is safer not to.

29 PICTURE CHARTS ASSIST THE LANGUAGE-IMPAIRED

Not if the Stroke has a receptive dysphasia, is agnosic (unable to recognize what the picture represents), if gestural communication is blitzed (nods for both yes and no) or is visually impaired.

Exception

They might. Get advice from the speech and language therapist first.

30 COMPENSATE FOR CURRENT DISABILITY

This is one of the reasons why the traditional 'generalist' approach to stroke rehabilitation, at any stage, is so unsuccessful.

This 'Why?' is a useful workshop question! Answers can be summarized as 'lack of neurological knowhow', exemplified in the confusion over current ability and future competence in which this particular method is rooted.

Working merely to improve performance of existing abilities excludes and denies or disrupts the use of ongoing natural recovery, the laying or relaying of alternative networking to replicate normal activity, and the learning or relearning of normal tasks.

Predictive assessment is crucial to the success of any rehabilitation programme, and generous allowances for future improvement must be inbuilt.

Exception

Measures which facilitate existing normal ability without endangering potential progress are, of course, wholly commendable.

31 THE NEUROLOGICAL APPROACH TO STROKE REHABILITATION TAKES LONGER AND IS UNNECESSARY FOR ELDERLY OR SEVERE STROKES

The next statement is usually: 'Functional activity is more important'.

Said by those who are unaware that the result of a stroke is purely neurological and therefore can only be 'neurologically' rehabilitated.

'Neurological rehabilitation' prevents the development of further disability, unmasks, re-educates and reinforces natural recovery, and facilitates – or relays alternative – neuronal networking to restore impaired function – and therefore gives everyone a chance to rehabilitate better and faster.

Any other approach will merely utilize existing ability (reflex patterns and all) and teach compensatory solutions (misusing all that lovely learning and re-learning ability) to assist the client merely to survive with ongoing disability.

Even severely impaired Strokes will improve sufficiently to enable easier and more comfortable management by others, which in turn improves quality of life and a sense of partnership in their own care.

As neurological rehabilitation programmes are rooted in pre-stroke normal functional abilities, it is the only genuinely functional approach. **The neurological approach is the functional approach!**

It is better to understand little than to misunderstand a lot.

(Anatole France)

PART THREE
'How'

Teamwork 9

For verily the tribe is all, and we are nothing singly save as parts of it.
(James Thomson)

In 1985 the World Health Organization published a list of targets for 'Health for All' by the year 2000:

> Target 29: By 1990, in all Member States, primary health care systems should be based on co-operation and teamwork between health personnel, individuals, families and community groups.... This could be achieved by policies in the countries that clearly define the role that different categories of health and social personnel should play in health care; basic, specialist and continuing education programmes for health personnel that provide insight, motivation and skill in inter-professional teamwork and in co-operation with individual families, groups and communities ...

Increasing knowledge about the complexities of CNS disablement indicates that traditional approaches to rehabilitation are no longer adequate. Not only do the professional rehabilitationists need to coordinate their programmes in order for the Stroke to achieve a return to maximal normality, but the partner or carer needs to be brought into the team too and, like the ripples spreading out in a pond, outer circles of friends, family, care assistants, support workers, etc. also need to be involved.

Two major issues deserve highlighting at this point. First, the centre of the circle is of course the Stroke, who in traditional medical models of care is excluded from the team altogether. A study by Partridge and Johnston (1989) found that patients with a higher level of perceived control over recovery made more progress with recovery from disability. The results showed that, in two groups of patients with very different disabilities (wrist fractures and hemiplegia following stroke) those who perceived more control over their rehabilitation recovered faster in both groups regardless of the initial severity. Patients recover better and faster when professionals accept them as partners in their own care.

Second, it is now recognized that genuine 'multidisciplinary' working increases the effectiveness of the rehabilitation programme because the input of each individual professional involved is reinforced and supported by the activities of the other members of the team.

In stroke rehabilitation the involvement of an extended team (to include the non-professionals working with the Stroke) is essential to re-establish those 'common denominators' of movement, communication, perception and social skills fundamental to all the activities of daily living.

This chapter discusses the need to define the term 'multidisciplinary' and offers some guidelines for the achievement of effective teamwork (certain sections are written in the first person plural as appropriate to professional colleagues):

9.1 Professional teamwork
9.2 Professional adulthood
9.3 The extended team
9.4 Common core skills

9.1 PROFESSIONAL TEAMWORK

Medical and other health care professionals are and always have been trained to be soloists, not members of an orchestra! We work alongside each other in a linear fashion; we serve no apprenticeship in partnering and therefore any overlapping instead of interlocking of our strengths and weaknesses can lead to tribal skirmishing or even war. The solution doesn't have to be a metamorphosis into a generic 'multitherapist', like a Peto Conductor for each condition, either. Every practitioner just has to learn to be complementary at work (Laidler, 1991).

There are many terms used to denote professional teamwork.

Transdisciplinary describes someone who works across the different professional borders, such as a keyworker or coordinator of services.

Multidisciplinary indicates that different disciplines are working with the same client towards the same long-term objective. It is an ambiguous term particularly in the UK where it is also understood to mean coordinated teamwork. It seldom does. The 'multidisciplinary approach' is a generic label which is applied to at least two other forms of patient care (Wilson and Laidler, 1990).

One is the **linear approach** (Figure 9.1); the traditional model where several disciplines work with the same patient, but from within their own professional boundaries and working practices. There is likely to be

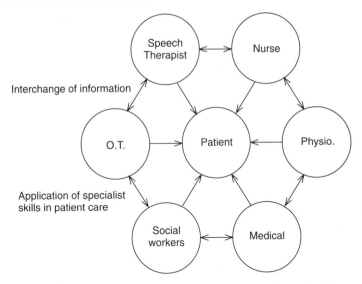

Figure 9.1 The linear approach in rehabilitation. (Reproduced with permission from Wilson, W.R. and Laidler, L.C.W., How teams can achieve 'skill-blend' in *Speech Therapy in Practice*.)

an exchange of information and ideas, but this has little effect on the essential clinical practice of each discipline involved.

The other is the **overlapping approach** (Figure 9.2), where members of different disciplines attempt to bridge professional boundaries by the uncritical sharing or poaching of each other's treatment techniques, which are then used without the educated selectivity of the original

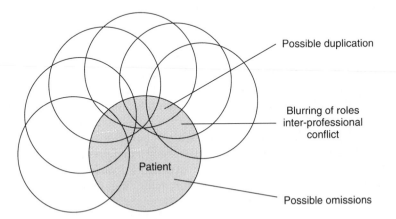

Figure 9.2 The overlapping 'grey area' approach to rehabilitation. (Reproduced with permission from Wilson, W.R. and Laidler, L.C.W., How teams can achieve 'skill-blend' in *Speech Therapy in Practice*.)

discipline. This can result in unnecessary duplications and/or omissions in treatment, and the indiscriminate and therefore often inappropriate application of techniques which may actually endanger progress. It also leads to a blurring or fragmentation of roles, the risk of interprofessional conflict, and confusion for clients, their families and other members of staff. In stroke rehabilitation these areas of overlap are known as the 'grey areas' of primary patient care.

'Interdisciplinary' implies the interwoven working together of different disciplines, but the process is frequently undermined in practice when applied to a particular patient or patient group because, just as in the 'multidisciplinary approach', there is no clearly-defined protocol to structure the integration of several disciplines into a seamless organism for a common purpose. However the term 'interdisciplinary' does afford a reasonably solid base on which to construct a model for professional teamwork.

This chapter refers to interdisciplinary working within the multi-disciplinary group. A definitive model is required in which:

- highly-specialized skills for each client group are developed within each professional discipline;
- specialized professionals cooperate effectively together.

There are two significant features which must be recognized if this is to be achieved.

Core expertise is basic to each qualified member of any profession as a core of knowledge specifically related to their professional training. To this is added ongoing clinical experience and postgraduate training concerning aspects of theory and practice within that profession and in related areas.

Skillblending is an inter-professional relationship in which the work of each professional is supported by – and in turn supports and reinforces – the work of others. This involves the judicious designation of – and education in – certain common core skills between the different professions which will enable a team to act as an integrated whole to achieve a truly holistic approach to rehabilitation. It is distinguishable from that uncritical sharing or poaching of techniques which characterizes the overlapping model. It is this skillblending which is the crux of good interdisciplinary teamworking, and it is perhaps the most difficult to achieve.

There are certain prerequisites for achieving an effective model. **Professional requirements** include:

- **balanced input**
  The team must include a Senior Clinician in each discipline who has the specialized knowledge appropriate to the client group.

- **accepted input**
  All the professionals within each discipline must be able and willing to recognize, acknowledge and respond to the core expertise of other professions.

- **comprehended input**
  Each team member must be familiar with the skills and concepts of the other team members in each discipline; this leads to a better understanding of the total picture of resources available to the client.

- **parameters of input**
  Team members must be able to identify those client needs which they themselves are not equipped to deal with. The responsibility then is to cross-refer.

- **coordinated input**
  Each team member must realize that it may be another member's role to initiate the activity in a specific area and to educate and advise others as appropriate, and each team member has to be willing and flexible enough to incorporate proposals from other professionals into their own treatment plan.

- **team management**
  A coordinator or teamleader should be identified to develop the corporate role of the team and to organize an adequate induction to new members. Junior members of each profession should be responsible to their senior colleagues clinically and to the team coordinator managerially.

- **general management**
  The senior specialist-clinicians should be jointly involved in the design and development of any management policies relating to the team and to the client group in which they are specializing. There must be common goals and shared strategies for intervention.

The **practical requirements** include:

- **communication network**
  (a) Formal
  Scheduled regular team meetings, in addition to case conference sessions, for the interchange of information (regarding treatment planning, client progress and goals, for instance), to update knowledge, and to introduce related areas of interest.
  (b) Informal
  The provision of an identified location or site where team members can meet in a more relaxed atmosphere, such as a shared staff-room. This can also facilitate the informal exchange of information and ideas on all aspects of specific skills and problems with client care.

  Good communication is essential for the development of an effective interdisciplinary team, and requires a considerable commitment in time set aside for this purpose by each of the professionals involved. This must be recognized as vital to the quality of client care.

- **joint workspace**
  If necessary in addition to the specific treatment areas required by each profession. This shared workspace provides opportunities for further communication and for team members to work together or consecutively with the same client, e.g. the speech therapist guiding the client's language skills, while the occupational therapist is progressing their executive skills; if the physiotherapist has just facilitated the client to gain and maintain automatic postural control in standing, the occupational therapist can immediately continue with a programme – for manual dexterity perhaps – involving standing to reinforce this. Shared workspace also gives ample time and facility for team members – including the client and family – to develop and guide each other through appropriate skillblending. In the case of residential clients, this workspace should be adjacent to their accommodation to maximize the nursing role in the team.

The **definitive interdisciplinary model** is one in which team members work in coordinate fashion, blending knowledge and skills to maximize the patient's potential for recovery.

Figure 9.3 highlights the essential difference between a team composed of many disciplines working in a disparate fashion and a truly interdisciplinary team.

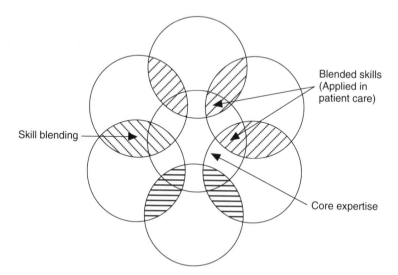

Figure 9.3 A definitive interdisciplinary model: effective rehabilitation. (Reproduced with permission from Wilson, W.R. and Laidler, L.C.W., How teams can achieve 'skill-blend' in *Speech Therapy in Practice.*)

The benefits of this model are graphically illustrated in Figure 9.4. This shows the changes in length of stay of patients on a stroke rehabilitation unit sampled at two stages during a four-year period. The dramatic difference in mean length of stay during these periods corresponded to periods during which very different approaches to patient care were employed. At the time of (**A**) the unit opened with a full complement of specialist senior clinicians and, with the exception of a named coordinator, operated in accordance with the guidelines described – the definitive interdisciplinary model. Two years on (**B**) and the mean length of stay had markedly increased. Interestingly, this difference in length of stay corresponds to a number of fundamental changes that could be observed in the structure of the rehabilitation team within the unit. Most significant among these changes were the loss of specialist senior staff and the actual physical relocation of the members of the team.

At the time sample (**B**) was taken, only two of the initially-appointed specialist senior clinicians remained in their posts. A new therapy chief could not recognize stroke rehabilitation as a specialty and this

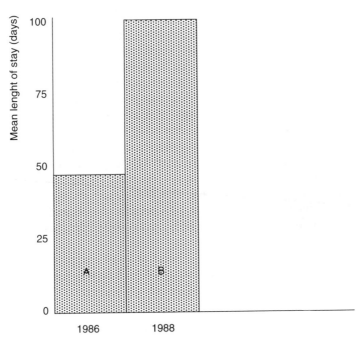

Figure 9.4 Difference in mean length of stay on a stroke unit under:
A, effective interdisciplinary management of stroke; and
B, unstructured 'traditional' management of stroke. (Reproduced with permission from Laidler, L.C.W., Adults – and how to become one in *Therapy Weekly*.)

influenced the commitment of the other service managers. Non-specialist senior staff were appointed to the unit, the structured induction programme for all new team members was discontinued and the status quo could not be regained. Further reorganization created changes in accommodation in the hospital within which the unit was based, and resulted in a loss of joint workspace and the recalling of disciplines to their geographically-distinct and widely-separated locations. Clinicians worked primarily in their own departments again, and this directly affected all aspects of team communication and skillblending. As a result, an overlapping approach to patient care plus the insular working practices characteristic of the linear model replaced the effective inter-disciplinary approach that had been achieved earlier. The criteria for selection of patients to, and their discharge from, the unit were adhered to throughout (Wilson and Laidler, 1990).

9.2 PROFESSIONAL ADULTHOOD

What divides men is less a difference in ideas than a likeness in pretensions.
(Pierre-Jean de Beranger)

Practical and professional pre-requisites for achieving the interdisciplinary ideal are necessary for the implementation of any policy, but the undercurrents from professional barriers run deep and are not so readily diverted. They can still disturb working relationships, whether intergroup or interpersonal, and are self-perpetuating unless we can track them to their source. It is relevant at this point to look a little deeper into ourselves instead of at each other in order to understand and relate our psychological infra-structure to team dynamics.

The concept of **adulthood** (Gilleard, 1992) described in Chapter 1 is a triad of autonomy, identity and engagement: autonomy, the spatial and temporal control of self; identity, the individual characteristics; and engagement, the facility to interact with people, objects and the environment. **Any one** of these elements can be voluntarily relinquished without loss of adulthood.

The attainment of personal adulthood enables competence in a professional (or any other) capacity, and it needs to be self-sustained as well as attributed, i.e. clearly recognized by oneself and others. If this concept is applied to a specifically-qualified group (doctors, nurses, therapists, etc.) then the triad of adulthood could be appropriately translated as:

autonomy	→	professional autonomy
identity	→	core expertise
engagement	→	attribution of responsibility (to and between self, clients, colleagues and carers)

and the group member would reflect this in their professional role. In this analogy of adulthood, by working as a member of a group of professional adults we are also accepting that by voluntarily sharing – or shelving or deferring – our professional autonomy we are **not** going to reduce – or lose – our professional adulthood.

It seems to be at this level that misunderstandings occur. The team is a collective of professional adults, but there is a reluctance to relinquish professional autonomies in a mixed team situation. It is this that leads to an ever-increasing elitism and the consequent collapse of holistic care. Attempts to overcome the problems without recognizing and remedying their cause frequently fail. This is illustrated in the 'overlapping' or 'grey area' approach (Figure 9.5), where members of different disciplines are each desperately hanging on to their respective professional autonomies while attempting to bridge professional barriers.

Possibly professional autonomy is thought to be an integral part of one's professional identity, and therefore there are very real fears of losing one's professional place altogether if it is reduced. But professional identity is our core expertise, which remains inviolate – as does our attribution of responsibility – so our professional adulthood is still intact. Furthermore, each member of the group retains their personal autonomy with which to determine a course of action, which could be to identify certain skills which can be shared, and to jointly select a coordinator to whom could be entrusted the various professional autonomies.

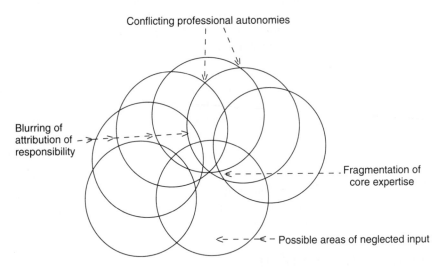

Figure 9.5 Conflicting areas in professional teamwork. (Reproduced with permission from Laidler, L.C.W., Adults – and how to become one in *Therapy Weekly*.)

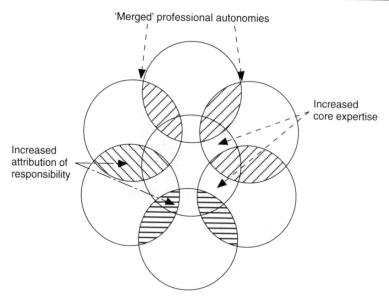

Figure 9.6 Professional adulthood in an interdisciplinary team. (Reproduced with permission from Laidler, L.C.W., Adults – and how to become one in *Therapy Weekly*.)

The positive way to ensure the balance of professional adulthood in this team situation, having voluntarily relinquished the separate professional autonomies, is for each member to increase their own core expertise (building greater specialist knowledge) and to update and broaden the areas of engagement/attribution of responsibility – referral and deferral to and from and between others.

> We trained hard...but it seemed that every time we were beginning to form up in teams, we would be reorganized. I was to learn later in life that we tend to meet any new situation by reorganizing – and a wonderful method it can be for creating the illusion of progress while producing confusion, inefficiency and demoralization.
>
> From the writings of Petronius Arbitor, Governor of Bithynia, who committed suicide in AD65.

Personal or professional suicide is not the solution to problems in professional teamwork, however! The solution lies instead in the definitive interdisciplinary model (Figure 9.6).

9.3 THE EXTENDED TEAM

Strokes are at maximum neurophysiological risk and maximum social disadvantage; professionally isolated and isolating practices cannot be pursued in these situations.

Repetitive or habitual activity exerts physiological stress which programmes and re-programmes motor behaviour (Chapter 3). This means that everyone bears the responsibility for enabling and disabling people who have sustained CNS trauma. Every time a Stroke is moved, positioned, handled and communicated with, normality or abnormality is actually being reinforced, i.e. if the same Stroke is approached and handled differently by members of health care teams, carers and family during each 24-hour period, this will create confusion in motor relearning and fail to reinforce the natural recovery or the spontaneous moments of normal activity; and if abnormal postures and movements are endorsed or incorporated into other actions in this way, then disability is being habituated.

In many instances the weight of caring is in the hands of unqualified or uninformed support workers and/or family members, and the significance of this rehabilitation factor is not even recognized. In these cases the stroke disabilities are compounded and the Stroke is denied any hope of recovering any aspect of further normality.

All people interacting with the Stroke form the extended team, including personal carers, family and close friends, who all have an advantage over the professionals in that they knew the Stroke before the disaster. Not only can they spot small but possibly significant changes that may have escaped even the most vigilant professional, but their involvement in the handling and rehabilitation programmes ensures that progress is maintained and acquired disability is contained.

There are of course exceptions to every rule! Some partners or families really do not know the Stroke as an individual very well, or are themselves unrealistic or uncaring about the outcome. Nevertheless, their inclusion into the team is still relevant if only to exclude the possibility of misjudgement or misunderstandings, and also to gauge the degree of support available – vitally important for realistic planning.

An extended team also generates more realistic appraisal and targetting of resources. Community networking is promoted with the inclusion of the family doctor, district nurses and outwork groups who will be responsible for ongoing care.

The listed practical prerequisites for professional teamworking can be adjusted to suit the inclusion of non-professional members. Time and space for skillblending for the learning of appropriate common core skills, joint assessments of current and predicted progress perhaps using a scheme like STARS in Chapter 5, shared therapy sessions to allow immediate carers and the Strokes to gain confidence in their own and each other's skills, and for formal and informal communication – such as acceptance into relevant case conferences, for instance, and relaxed discussion – are needed to bring the whole business of stroke into a normal everyday perspective.

9.4 COMMON CORE SKILLS

These are, in effect, all concerned with normal functional activity. This of course covers the whole 24 hours of every day to include nighttime positioning in bed and turning, drinks and medication and toilet needs.

Dynamic postural control against gravity is fundamental to all activity, and is undoubtedly the major (and often the most disregarded) impairment following a stroke. To regain this is the paramount objective in stroke rehabilitation. Without it, even unimpaired physical and cognitive structuring of motor behaviour cannot produce an unflawed movement. It is also impossible for the Stroke to regain this dynamic control without informed intervention (unless the stroke resulted in insignificant impairment).

The relevant professional skills need to be recognized and explored so that common core skills can be identified, shared and implemented by everyone living or working with the Stroke (including night-staff), in order to gain and reinforce and sustain progress.

These common core skills encompass:

- communication;
- positioning;
- handling;
- dressing and undressing (and selection of clothes);
- feeding and eating;
- getting into and out of bed, including coping with bedclothes;
- on and off the toilet, with rearrangement of clothing before and after, and wiping and hand-washing;
- getting from sitting to standing, and from standing to sitting;
- walking or wheelchair management;
- manoeuvring into positions appropriate for further activity.

Advice on ways and means is given in the next chapter.

Nine-tenths of wisdom is being wise in time.

(Theodore Roosevelt)

REFERENCES

Gilleard, C.J. (1992) Losing one's mind and losing one's place: a psychosocial model of dementia, in *Gerontology: Responding to an Ageing Society* (ed. K. Morgan), British Society of Gerontology, Jessica Kingsley, London.

Laidler, L.C.W. (1990) Adults – and how to become one. *Therapy Weekly*, **17**(35), 4.

Laidler, L.C.W. (1991) Great expectations: multidisciplinary teamwork in practice. World Confederation for Physical Therapy Congress paper, publication pending in *Physiotherapy*.

Partridge, C.J. and Johnston, M. (1989) Perceived control of recovery from physical disability: measurement and prediction. *British Journal of Clinical Psychology*, **28**, 53–9.

Wilson, W.R. and Laidler, L.C.W. (1990) How teams can achieve 'skill-blend'. *Speech Therapy in Practice*, 7–8.

Rehabilitative strategies

10

Boast not thyself of tomorrow; for thou knowest not what a day may bring forth.

(Old Testament, Book of Proverbs, xxvii: 1)

Rehabilitation of stroke, of course, needs to be started at once to ensure that the preventable problems – such as spasticity and the physiological 'learning' of abnormal function and non-use (or over-use) of existing abilities – do not override the recovery process. However, therapeutic intervention at any stage – even years after the event – can effectively reduce these problems even if they are already programmed in, but much greater physiological stressing is required and some consequences such as damaged or osteoporotic joints and soft tissue contractions may be irreversible.

Natural recovery in the first few days or weeks is misleading in that it can be accounted for by the resolution of acute inflammation and/or oedema around the site of the lesion.

Further recovery can be attributed to:

- spontaneous reorganization (more often in less significant lesions) where acquired disability has been prevented (or not acquired!);
- acquired reorganization resulting from rehabilitative intervention.

In the early stages, relearning and the absorption of natural recovery proceeds in an apparently haphazard fashion: one function is perhaps reaching a plateau as CNS reorganization takes place, while several others may be leapfrogging forwards (or backwards, if guidance is withheld). The need for appropriate interception is paramount throughout (like a juggler spinning plates on sticks), otherwise the momentum gets lost and any progression or 'carry-over' of ability halts or becomes subverted.

Attempting to pick up where the last visit ended – or to form detailed plans for ongoing treatments – is a worthless exercise in the early stages of stroke rehabilitation because the picture and the problem changes continuously. Variable external and internal factors account for this unpredictability and it is only clinical experience and instinct that can forecast – and then only very broadly – the responses of the Stroke to the known factors which affect performance.

In the later stages of rehabilitation, some of these factors can be deliberately introduced into formal therapy sessions in preparation for the 'munch-crunch' reality of home and community life – but only when the Stroke can take them on without adverse repercussions.

External factors influencing rehabilitation include:

- **management**
  Poor or irregular positioning and handling and inactivity between formal sessions creates confusion in motor learning and relearning, and reinforces disability. Common core skills are explored in section 10.2.
- **climate**
  A cold environment reduces the elasticity of muscle tissue, and slows circulatory activity; hypertonicity and spasticity are therefore increased. Conversely, undue warmth lowers muscle tone, but also reduces the stimulation levels in neurologically-impaired muscles. Both hypertonic and hypotonic states need to put in more effort to initiate and complete movement, which can then trigger reflex activity and increase spasticity. Most Strokes find that moving or sustaining posture against gravity is extra tiring in these circumstances. ('It's cold enough to wear a stick!', Peter Cranfield, stroke-survivor, struggling in for a coffee in mid-winter.)
- **clothing**
  Extra warmth can be provided by 'thermal' quality mittens and socks for S hands and feet. Restrictive clothing restricts physical activity. Overloose garments can twist or slip and can hide abnormal – or complicate normal – movement patterns.
- **footwear**
  As above!
- **environment**
  Noise and interruption distracts. Floors, if slippery, increase anxiety and reduce performance; if carpeted this requires extra agility in locomotion, and loose mats or rugs create hazards.

Internal factors: any personal tension enhances hypertonic and reflexive movement and affects concentration; if performance appears poor and unaccounted for by external factors, then observation and/or enquiry may elicit other reasons, such as:

- **anxiety**
  This can be personal or about others, natural or pathological, episodic or longer-lasting.

- **pain**
  From traumatized joints, abdominal distension, local inflammation (pressure areas, cuts and bruises) constipation, urinary retention, etc.
- **fatigue**
  From poor or disturbed sleep, over-activity, inadequate nutrition, infection or other pathological conditions such as anaemia.
- **ill-health**
  Respiratory distress, cardiac inefficiency, infection (cystitis, pneumonia, etc), thrombophlebitis, a cold, etc.
- **malnutrition**
  A particular risk with dysarthric and dysphagic Strokes, and for others, also, for these reasons:
  - inadequate diet;
  - help with feeding may not be offered, and slow eaters may not be given time to finish;
  - unacceptable foods (on religious/ethnic/personal or medical dietary grounds);
  - previous or newly presenting digestive tract conditions;
  - depressed appetite (due to urine retention, faecal impaction, depression, etc.);
  - other disease processes.

A nutritional study of 100 patients in a psychogeriatric unit – which also included young patients for assessment – demonstrated that despite dietetic and managerial strategies designed to improve nutritional status (one of the diet supplements was costing the service an extra £11,000 a year in 1986) 35% showed a deficiency in Vitamin C, 8% had red blood cell folates below normal levels, 24% had low levels of serum Vitamin D, and many were seriously underweight (Fenton, 1989). This indicates the importance of recognizing these other factors.

It is important to bear in mind also that the normal ageing process – and the possible development of other pathological disease processes – continues throughout the post-stroke rehabilitation period, and also that chronic physical disability may be due more to a cognitive constraint than physical constraints: cognition is the mediator of motor performance.

The one factor that does remain constant (except possibly in Alzheimer's disease) is learning ability. Cognitive and motor programming and re-programming only ends with life itself. Underlying all the theory and practice now should be recognition of the neurological cause of dysfunction following stroke, and of the all-important factor of neuromuscular plasticity.

The core expertise of each profession includes many different approaches to the rehabilitation of stroke, and controversy over techniques within and between professional groups tends to add to an already inherent tendency to overlook the basic – and vital – issues. 'Techniques' are not for general application to all Strokes, but can be gainfully employed with some. These are specialized forms of intervention, however, and need expert 'live' tuition, so none of them are described here. In their place is the basic premise introduced by the Bobaths, which gives a pragmatic concept from which to build an effective repertoire of strategies for implementation:

> Rehabilitation is based on the handling of the patient to give back to that person inhibitory control over their abnormal patterns of movement and to enable a normal, or relearned normal, response.

This approach could be criticized as being too heuristic, but rehabilitation is of necessity largely heuristic. Research programmes are slowly validating or disproving certain modalities, but this is retrospective on existing methods. Developments in the field of rehabilitation are rooted in scientific theorizing and clinical reasoning, particularly with regard to CNS trauma.

The strategies described in this chapter are those which have utilized the newer knowledge, and been developed and evaluated in clinical practice with effective teamwork and excellent results: remarkably good functional and psychological recovery has been gained and maintained in even the most severe Strokes.

The ways and means are deliberately general and applicable in both professional and domestic situations. The successful outcome depends entirely on the holistic approach throughout, which provides the steady rehabilitative foundation upon which further specific professional input can build improvements to particular components. Rehabilitation of stroke is a 'hands on' process; recovery is (almost literally) moulded until the Stroke can personally sustain and maintain it.

The major maxims arising from the previous chapters include:

- the simple equations on which to base practical clinical methods for regaining dynamic balance and functional movement:
  CoG = centre of gravity (see Chapter 2);
  BoS = base of support (that which supports the body against gravity: feet, thighs/chair, etc.);
  CoG over BoS = stability;
  CoG – BoS = instability;
  CoG : BoS, the controlled movement of CoG relative to BoS = mobility + stability = functional movement.
- dynamic postural control anticipates and allows freedom of peripheral limb movement.
- normal movement generates normal movement – it opens and re-opens pathways and introduces auto-initiated (natural) control of inhibition and excitation. So to facilitate normal movement is to launch an ongoing process towards normality.

- gross patterns of movement precede fragmented components of movement.
- familiar and task- and context-specific actions can prompt a natural and spontaneous follow-through and can also re-lay the rules to assist response selection for 'carry-over' into other activities.
- stressing, in the physiological sense of repetition over a period of time, reinforces plastic adaptation.
- controlled environmental factors help to ensure stability and continuity for the rehabilitation process.

Clinical reasoning is fundamental to the creation of strategies, and involves an assessment and analysis of the presenting problems at each contact episode of care that relies on a working knowledge of normal movement patterns and their underlying neuromuscular derivation.

It is necessary to utilize the basic means of positioning, handling and facilitation throughout. These are of course an almost indivisible and continuous process, but are subsectioned here for revision. Because of the quantity of advice on offer the chapter is divided into two portions for easier digestion:

10.1 Positioning
10.2 Handling
10.3 Common Core Skills

contain general information applicable to the rehabilitation of all Strokes.

Everyone – all professional disciplines as well as support workers and personal carers – working with stroke survivors should be practised in and prepared to assist the Stroke in these areas. The same methods apply to all other activities of daily living, to enable each Stroke to regain dynamic postural control as early as possible – this is the first and most vital step in rehabilitation – and maximum functional independence as soon as possible.

Detailed procedures for the therapeutic assistance of the major everyday activities – washing, dressing and undressing, toileting, oral feeding and getting on and off the floor – are described in Chapter 13.

10.4 Special
10.5 Practical strategies
10.6 Specific problems
10.7 Predictive assessment

give more specialized guidance and suggestions for some specific problem-solving.

The procedures are all presented for use with early or severely-disabled Strokes, and progressive strategies outlined or deemed obvious.

The reader can modify or extend the input required relative to the performance and ability of each individual.

10.1 POSITIONING

The concept of reflex inhibition underlies the preparation for – and the accomplishment of – all movement following a stroke. Controlled positioning, therefore, is a basic strategy from the very beginning.

Furniture should be arranged in such a way that all activity is to the S side, i.e. lockers and tables to the S side of the bed or chair, and the getting in and out of bed is done to the S side.

If hemianopia or unilateral neglect is pronounced, attention can be focused initially to the centre front: consistent prompting to encourage the necessary turning to the S side will give a kick-start to the rehabilitation of this problem.

IN BED

The mattress and pillows support the entire length of the body, giving the maximum BoS. Lying, turning and rolling, and coming up to the sitting position with legs over the side of the bed should be carried out to both sides, but mostly to the S side, to ensure normal and dynamic weight-bearing activity through the proximal joints (hips and shoulders) of the body and natural rotation between thorax and pelvis.

Supine lying (on one's back) is not to be encouraged – it exacerbates reflex retraction of the S shoulder girdle, with adduction, flexion and internal rotation of the arm (usually clutched across the chest), slight flexion at the hip and lateral rotation of the leg (the cause of pressure sores over the lateral malleolus) with plantarflexion and inversion of the foot. To prevent this, pillows need to be placed lengthways under the S side of the body, from scapula to knee (Figure 10.1).

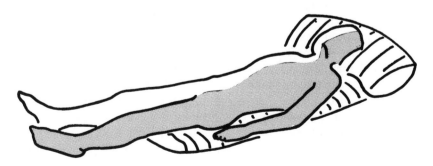

Figure 10.1 Supported supine lying.

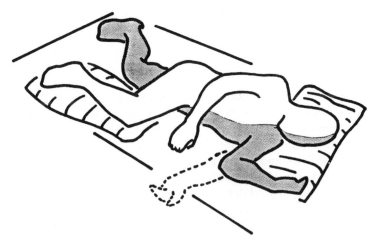

Figure 10.2 Lying on the S side.

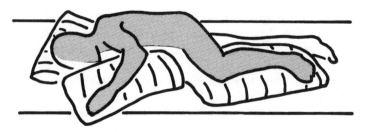

Figure 10.3 Lying on the N side.

Lying on the S side should be encouraged, with the S shoulder well forward (protracted) so that the body weight is supported on the flat of the scapula to prevent pressure on the vulnerable glenohumeral joint (Figure 10.2), and to maintain a little rotation and elongation in the trunk muscles. This frees the N arm to reach for articles on bedside lockers, etc: each reach will subtly 'roll' weight over the proximal joints for early dynamic postural reactions. The S leg should be in mid-line extension at the hip and slight flexion at the knee.

When lying on the N side, pillows may be required to support the weight and maintain correct position of the S limbs: arm well forward with scapula protracted, and leg with slight flexion at hip and knee (Figure 10.3). Make sure that there's plenty of room between the body and the edge of the bed (on both sides!) and that the Stroke is aware of this factor in order to relearn and relate spatial awareness and judgement to personal space and safety. Teach the Stroke to reach for and feel for edges (and **not** to pull on them), and to 'sweep' surfaces between their body and edges with their hands to reinforce spatial parameters.

Bedrails and cotsides, 'monkey-poles' (overbed pulley) and rope ladder systems for pulling the body up into sitting positions are **not** for Stroke use. Any grabbing and pulling action triggers the grasp and upper limb reflexes and increases extensor tone as the trunk musculature takes up the strain to support the muscles of the shoulder girdle to protect the glenohumeral joint. Pulling on the cotside or the edge of the bed does not assist the forward roll or sitting up; it actually initiates extension away from the desired goal. In addition the effort involved in overcoming this extensor response unleashes abnormal reflex activity, and the strongly-sustained protraction of the N arm enforces retraction and hypertonus of the musculature of the S shoulder and trunk (try this as a workshop exercise).

Only put up a protective cotside when a Stroke with severe unilateral neglect, anosodiaphoria or anosognosia – or who is hyperactive or disorientated – is in bed and unattended. These are the Strokes who are at risk of rolling out, falling out or even leaping out of bed regardless. The difficulty then is to dissuade the Stroke from using the cotsides continuously as convenient grab-rails.

Bony protuberances need protection while the Stroke remains inactive, or when hyper-reflexia or 'spasms' are poorly controlled. Fleecy pieces of material (man-made are easier to wash than genuine sheepskin) placed across the bed under the lower leg help to prevent heel and ankle sores developing: a full-length piece will protect the full length of the body. Made into short tubes (with the stitching and seams on the outside) and worn over the elbows, it will protect from over-use friction; in the shape of a bootee (seams outside) it will protect the hyperactive Stroke even better than a piece of fleece in the bed. If skin is broken or looks inflamed and soggy, seek guidance from nurses and notify the doctor.

IN SITTING

Here the BoS is decreased (now from the toetips of the feet on the floor to the point of contact of the trunk or head on the back of the chair; if leaning forward, to the back of the rump on the chairseat).

Gravity is exerting force on any unsupported sections of the body, and this is extremely tiring for neurologically-impoverished musculature. No Stroke should be expected to sit and remain alert and untroubled in this situation for long periods. If tiredness is apparent, then a short rest lying down (in a therapeutic position on the bed) will prevent abnormal postures developing and provide an extra exercise – getting on and off the bed in the prescribed manner (section 10.2) a few times a day is itself a rehabilitation strategy!

However, if the Stroke is seated leaning back and fully-supported (Figure 10.4) for most of the day, then the normal anti-gravity systems

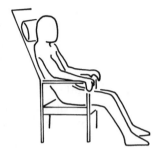

Figure 10.4 Lying back fully-supported for long periods weakens postural musculature (through disuse) and disorganizes the righting reflex.

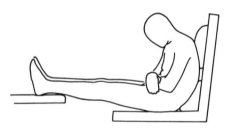

Figure 10.5 Lengthy slump sitting weakens muscles by impoverishing innervation.

are not operating. Once these are lost through infrequent use – and the vestibular system re-programmed to accept leaning back as normal erect posture (so that really upright feels like falling forwards) – re-education is a long, frightening and arduous process.

A second important factor is that prolonged 'slump' sitting (Figure 10.5) impoverishes innervation to all muscles, resulting in generalized weakness.

Instead of the low-slung long-backed support chairs traditionally provided, short-upright-backed armchairs, or dining-type chairs with arms, should be used; they should be of sufficient height that knees and

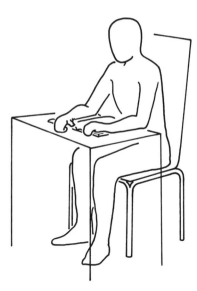

Figure 10.6 Sitting comfortably: a recommended position.

hips can be right-angled and both feet can rest on the floor. With the head, neck, shoulders and upper trunk unsupported in sitting, natural control against gravity is stimulated and sustained from the start. The most effective sitting position is leaning forward with both arms resting on a table in front (Figure 10.6). It is also useful for reading, drinks and meals, is sociable too, and if returning to bed for a rest is impractical then a pillow on the table that the head can be rested upon is an option.

Sitting for long in one position is unnatural and for Strokes who have difficulty in wriggling or shifting periodically to another position it is important that they are assisted to do so – it's all part of the rehabilitation process. As in lying, body weight needs to be distributed naturally through alternate sides of the body and through the proximal joints (hips and shoulders). The pressure areas of heavy or inactive people need protection, too: a fleece to sit on is sometimes sufficient. For longer use, one of the many purpose-designed cushions may be necessary. Seek advice from therapists and nurses.

Ensure that the Stroke is able to sit in the chair with his or her rump well back against the junction between seat and back – short thighs, long seats, too high a chair without a footstool or too many cushions result in sitting with the rump to the front of the seat and a long lean backwards for support against the chairback (which reinforces underlying extensor reflexia and postural weakness). It is usually these people who persistently slither out of their chairs. Prevent this happening by making sure that the chair fits the person, and that the rump is established well back into the chair to give right-angled flexion at the hips. If the problem continues, reinforce and increase hip flexion by:

- providing a lower chair;
- putting a wedge-cushion behind their back, thin end down;
- placing a wedge-cushion under the seat-cushion – or under the thighs – wide end to the front.

The **S arm** must be comfortably supported so that pressure is transmitted up from the elbow to accurately approximate the glenohumeral joint and also to stimulate peripheral inhibition of abnormal tone and movement, with the wrist level or slightly extended and fingers relaxed. Use a pillow(s) or cushion(s) from the arm of the chair to the lap if a table isn't available.

Concentrate on symmetry for some of the time (maintaining a totally static position isn't normal! See Chapter 8), and ask all passers-by to check limb positions – that the S foot is never resting in the inverted and/or plantar-flexed position (Figure 10.7), and that the S arm isn't dangling or trapped.

Encourage the Stroke to sit for some of the time with their palms together and fingers interlaced – this helps to maintain a functional position of slight extension at the wrist with the metacarpo-phalangeal

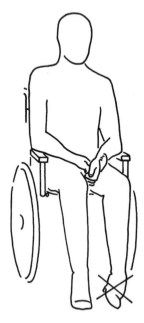

Figure 10.7 Keep a constant check on the hands and feet.

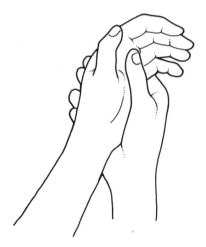

Figure 10.8 Comfortable, corrective and supportive hold for S hand.

(MCP) joints semi-flexed and comfortably spaced. Assist the hands into this position if necessary, as struggling increases the difficulties. Advise the Stroke to start at the heel of the S hand, and gently slide the fingers of the N hand up the S palm into the webs between the S fingers until both hands are comfortably clasped.

If spasticity is already pronounced in the S hand, demonstrate the alternative (Figure 10.8): cradling the S wrist in the N hand, N thumb lying up the S palm to the MCP joints to maintain S wrist partly supinated and in slight extension. Advise the use of this 'self-help' hold during transfers etc., and use it for all general mobilizing when both hands need to be 'linked'. This saves time and gives confidence – clasped hands usually end up screwed up – and the knowledge that the N hand can be quickly disentangled for emergency use is very comforting.

Mobilizing with tightly-interlinked fingers reduces concentration on the mobilizing itself because processing of sensory information from the hands and fingers has a very high profile in the CNS (try it – it's distracting).

WHEN PUSHING PEOPLE IN WHEELCHAIRS

Make certain that both feet are placed on the footplates, and ensure that the S foot is **not** scooped up to rest – inverted and plantarflexed – across the N ankle, even for a few yards. It's a nasty habit and instantly establishes the S leg as a passenger instead of a necessary limb, as well as reinforcing the abnormal pattern.

10.2 HANDLING

Handling is a keyword in stroke rehabilitation. It is the factor linking everyone – professional, non-professional and family – working or living with a stroke-survivor at any stage. It is integral to the recovery of independence in all the activities of everyday life.

Skilled handling enables and escalates a return to normality; inept handling creates confusion and reinforces disablement.

Handling incorporates proprioceptive prompting, cueing (gestural clues) and/or physically assisting the Stroke to make every move as normal as possible. This applies to all parts of the body – limbs, trunk and head postures – and to the ongoing sequences until the move is completed, and is fundamental to the recovery of natural performance.

Always work from and to the Stroke-affected side, and slightly in front if relevant to the occasion (if the Stroke has a tendency to fall forwards, or has marked visual field defects or severe unilateral neglect).

Establish eye contact on approach before starting any procedure. Ensure eyes follow and maintain awareness, if appropriate, of any actions. Encourage concentration until the Stroke displays signs of fatigue, then stop for a rest or change to a new activity to re-stimulate interest. Relaxed reciprocation is all that is required from the Stroke; effort should be confined to the helper! Effort by the Stroke increases reflex activity and immediately distorts normal performance. Never say, 'Try', or, 'Try harder', it actually makes everything more difficult for everybody.

MOBILITY IN BED

Turning, rolling, moving across the bed and up to the pillows are all simple moves that need skilled handling to promote early independence. **Moving across the bed** incorporates 'bridging' – raising the pelvis just clear of the sheets without allowing the extending hips to trigger reflex extensor thrust in the S leg. Assist the S knee to bend in order to bring both knees into flexion ('crook' lying) with feet flat on bed. If necessary support (or sit on!) the S foot to keep it in position. Pulling the knees/thighs forward over the feet will help to initiate the bottom-lifting action for the shift to either side. However, 'bridging' as an exercise when it is **not** part of another movement will only reinforce these reflexes – don't do it!

To turn on to the N side, the S knee can be helped into flexion, the S shoulder guided forwards and the S arm supported to reach forwards; this starts trunk rotation and alignment (righting reactions) so that the pelvis rolls naturally into the side-lying position on the S side with S hand ready to support on the bed (Figure 10.9).

For turning on the S side, the helper stands on the S side facing the oncoming roll. Remove obstructive bedclothes and guide the N arm and

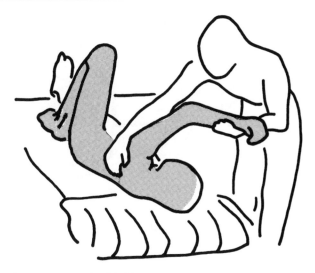

Figure 10.9 Rolling over to the N side.

shoulder over the body in the direction of the turn as before (Figure 10.10). The N hand is guided to support the body on the bed to prevent rolling off (Figure 10.11), and is then in place to assist the push up into a sitting position as both legs swing over the edge of the bed – if this is the next planned move (Figure 10.12).

Lying-to-sitting should be a fluid counterbalancing procedure: reverse it for getting back to lie down on the bed (and vice versa to get up to the N side). However, always try to ensure that getting in and out of bed is to the **S side** – to maintain self-inhibitory control over primitive reflexia and to stimulate supporting reactions in the S arm.

For moving up the bed, encourage the Stroke to turn on to the N side with knees and hips flexed, rise up to take weight on the N forearm, and

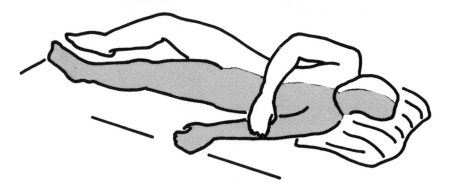

Figure 10.10 Rolling to the S side.

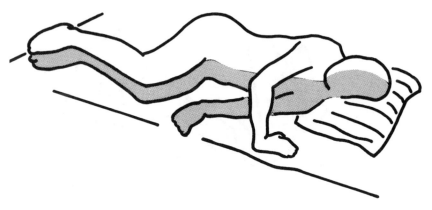

Figure 10.11 Up from lying on the S side.

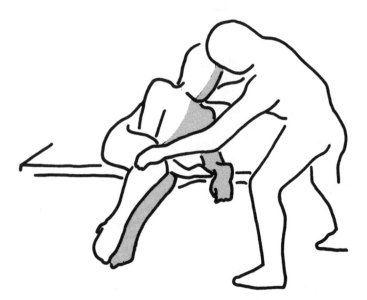

Figure 10.12 Up to sit on the side of the bed.

shunt towards the pillows using feet for push (keeping knees flexed). If this triggers extension reflex patterns, go for sitting on the edge of the bed to the S side, feet on floor, helper in front (bracing the Stroke's knees with own knees, both hands behind the Stroke's shoulders), and facilitate the individual to shunt up the side of the bed by part-rising clear of the bed and re-sitting again nearer the goal – until the bottom is in the appropriate place – before lying down again.

TRANSFERS

These are the assisted moves from a sitting position to another seat: between a bed and a chair; to a commode or lavatory; between wheel-chair and chair; or into a seat in a vehicle. The next seat should be placed at a right angle to the starting position wherever possible.

Never lift under the S shoulder or pull the S arm: this traumatizes the glenohumeral joint.

The swivel transfer encourages active participation. Practise it first yourself, keeping CoG over bent knees, swinging your bottom between the two seats without moving feet (but allowing them to swivel as the body swivels) to judge the natural placing of the feet – roughly mid-way between the seats – and demonstrate this actively to the Stroke before starting. Hands are not required; this is all postural trunk and lower limb control, so the S hand can be linked or supported with the N hand.

For a transfer to the S side, the helper stands in front of the S side, nearside foot on the inside of the S foot to maintain slight lateral eversion, and knee just alongside the lateral aspect of the S knee (much easier than it sounds). The nearside arm supports around (with pressure into) the thorax under the N arm, and the outside arm cradles the S shoulder girdle over the S arm to exert lifting pressure into the scapular region, but not gripping the scapula itself (Figure 10.13).

The Stroke should have plenty of space in which to come forward, bringing the CoG over the feet, as the helper pulls forwards and up;

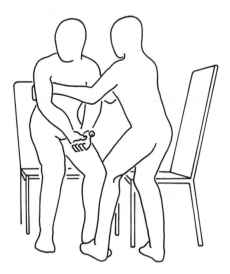
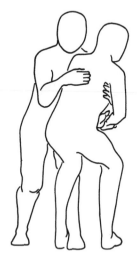

Figure 10.13 The swivel transfer.

helper's head leaning away to the N side as the Stroke's head comes forwards into the gap over the helper's outside shoulder.

Don't let the Stroke stand fully upright with straightened knees – this gets into an unstable transfer involving much shuffling of feet and difficulty in controlling the fully-erect Stroke teetering on a small BoS (two feet, one of them unreliable).

Instead, with all the knees still slightly flexed, the helper swings the Stroke through the 90° turn and into the second seat, keeping the CoG well over the feet until the Stroke is re-seated.

For transfers to the N side, the helper's outside knee and foot controls the S leg.

For grabbers and pullers, insist that the Stroke holds something in the N hand (preferably their S hand (Figure 10.14) or a handkerchief, a notebook ... anything except bits of the helper (or the arm of the chair they are moving from).

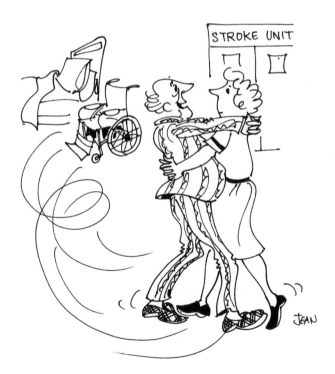

DID YOU SAY 'HANG ON AND PIVOT'?

Do explain first!

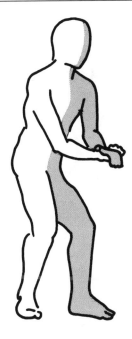

Figure 10.14 Grabbers and pushers must hold something in their N hand.

TO STANDING

The move from sitting to standing takes the CoG from over the large BoS (the area from where the trunk rests against the back of the chair to the tips of the toes on the floor) to a small BoS (the two feet). Always initiate the move by guiding the Stroke to lean forwards (gentle pressure between the shoulder blades or behind the shoulders), to bring the CoG over the feet.

If the Stroke has been sitting with bottom well into the back of the seat, then assisted 'hip-walking' (Figure 10.15) – weight transference from buttock to buttock – will achieve the necessary advance of weight to the front edge of the seat. The feet have often tucked under automatically by this time; if not, then the helper needs to guide them backwards to provide the BoS for the next move – the method as for a swivel transfer but without the swivel! – allowing the Stroke to complete the initial rising to an upright standing position with straightened knees.

Frail or arthritic Strokes will want to make use of any available support. When they are able to control their balance themselves, just assist the above move but allow them to push up from the arms of the chair (Figure 10.16) rather than pull on the helper (but check with the physiotherapist first).

Ensure that the S foot is flat on the floor; the helper's nearside foot will have prevented inversion at the S ankle, and judicious pressure from the helper's nearside knee can establish or prompt extension of the S knee.

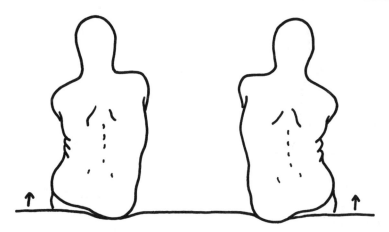

Figure 10.15 'Hip-walking' to the front of the seat prior to rising.

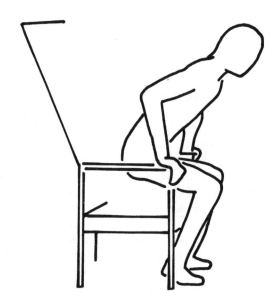

Figure 10.16 Pushing up from the arms of a chair.

Pressure downwards on the S side of the pelvis by the helper's outside hand reinforces S heel contact with the floor if necessary, and the backwards swing of hyper-reflexive trunk musculature can also be controlled from the pelvis or shoulders with the same hand.

10.3 COMMON CORE SKILLS

The common core skills are those needed to accomplish the carry-over of specific professional input into the everyday performance of functional activity. They are rooted in handling and communication strategies (which initiate active responses) to promote an early return to dynamic balance control and social confidence, ensure progress and maximize independence. They require the explicit sharing of all the relevant knowledge relating to, and implicit in, all routine activities:

- turning and moving in bed, coping with bedclothes;
- getting in and out of bed, coping with bedclothes;
- standing up and sitting down;
- going to the lavatory and coping with clothing and cleaning;
- washing, dental hygiene (tooth-brushing, dentures);
- dressing, hair care;
- feeding;
- transfers;
- reaching and turning;
- walking, steps, stairs, opening doors, manoeuvring around obstacles, turning round;
- getting up from (and down onto) the floor;
- wheelchair management;

The specific expertise required in these everyday activities is contributed by:

- dieticians: nutritional status; nutritional needs.
- doctors: clinical condition; medication and side-effects.
- family/friends/carers: personal knowledge; expectations and needs.
- nurses: continence; pressure areas; day-/nighttime behaviour.
- occupational therapists: activities of daily living; perceptual problems; aids to independence.
- physiotherapists: normal and abnormal movement; facilitation of movement; walking aids.
- psychologists: cognitive state; social behaviours.
- social workers: social and financial factors; family expectations.
- speech and language therapists: verbal/written communication; gestural communication; communication needs and aids; feeding/swallowing problems.
- the stroke-survivor: expectations; preference/choices; personal strategies.

All these professionals, as well as non-professional carers, are likely to be involved with the Stroke in some or all of the activities of daily living and should be using the common core skills required in each activity. Dressing, for instance, includes undressing – and the appropriate assistance will be necessary not only for the top-to-toe procedure, but also in the taking-off and putting-on of outer garments between visits to other departments or clinic situations, and, of course, in every trip to the lavatory. Never forget the underlying principle of neuromuscular plasticity – **continuity of procedure is fundamental to stroke rehabilitation.**

The inclusion of family carers from the beginning – especially into the hospital ward – will help to establish familiar routines and awareness of ongoing improvements. It will also relieve pressure on staffing levels: professional input, after initial demonstration, can be further utilized in the sharing and monitoring of skills to ensure progressive rehabilitation.

The team input could include the following expertise:
- The nurses offer guidance on the management of continence, catheters, pressure areas, special needs such as support hose and any risk factors such as an unstable cardiac condition or blood pressure.
- The OT can recommend the order and manner of getting into and out of clothing, and advise upon or provide adaptations to garments such as velcro to replace zips and buttons and front-opening bras (or elastic across the gap for pulling on over the head to obviate the struggle to do up hooks and eyes).
- The physiotherapist can advise on ways to progress dynamic balance, to inhibit hyper-reflexia and spasticity, to facilitate normal limb movement and to control oedema.
- The speech therapist will advise on feeding, the use of communication charts or aids, clueing to encourage production of meaningful sound, specific programmes to rebuild grammatical construction and language and gestural communication systems.
- Family and friends can ensure loving support, links with the real world, the reassurance of identity and individuality and personal and appropriate clothing.
- The Stroke will demonstrate personal problems as they arise, and also personal choices and strategies (which may be better than those proffered!).

The therapeutic procedure for assisted washing, dressing and toileting is described step-by-step in Chapter 13.

It has been suggested that getting fully dressed while standing unsupported (including socks/tights and buckling or lacing-up shoes) is the ultimate test for balance! The most educational preparation for assisting functional activity is to try the activity out for oneself first. The perceptual and balance impairments cannot be simulated, but the physical

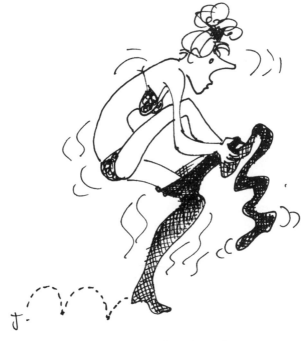

The ultimate test for balance?

actions involved when an arm and a leg on one side are (imagined to be) unco-ordinated or non-functioning should be experienced. Work through the sample list of daily routine activities given earlier in this section, first with one side inactive and then with the other. (Teeth-brushing and bottom-wiping, for instance, using the non-dominant hand, are particularly difficult even for the unhandicapped.)

It is important for the Stroke that daily routine activities are clearly understood to be therapeutic and as such are not subjected to rigid timekeeping (except in individually-customized bladder retraining programmes):

> *Never have I been more aware than in these last months how life-preserving my routine is. The day becomes a series of stepping-stones – from breakfast to household chores … so the routine makes a frame and I feel that there is a next stepping-stone … learn to take the chores as an exercise, deliberately slowing down, savouring … the making of order as delightful in itself – not just something to get out of the way.*
>
> *(May Sarton, 1988)*

Give time for relearning, coping and confidence. Wash and dress after breakfast if necessary. Skilfully facilitated, this is a more comprehensive, sophisticated and therapeutic 'exercise' than many of the non-context-specific treatments in a clinical setting; it involves rolling, turning and reaching, sitting and standing, and balance reactions throughout, and achieves faster results, too. And a properly-facilitated trip to the loo (Chapter 13) is just as rehabilitative as half-an-hour in a therapy department spent practising weight-transference in standing (could it even be a more beneficial alternative?).

10.4 SPECIAL SKILLS

Here it is appropriate to paraphrase Kidd (1992), with 'therapy' and 'therapist' replacing 'physiotherapy' and 'physiotherapist' in the original article:

> To perform on the neuromuscular system an episode of therapy should have such consequence of plastic adaptation that subtle differences in subsequent episodes are required ... A therapy which brings about a plastic adaptation of the neuromuscular system – requires a different therapy approach to bring about further plastic adaptations – which requires a different therapy approach...The therapy which initiates and directs the plastic adaptation of the neuromuscular system demands a continuously varying therapy approach.

In practical terms the therapist is actually a facilitator or enabler and, in many procedures from here on, will share the term 'helper' with all and sundry to simplify the text. It is naturally assumed that specialized skills and core expertise are being applied specifically to upgrade performance in the problem areas for each Stroke in addition to the following grassroot precepts:

- Cultivate heightened awareness of own and others' normal motor behaviour and relate it to individual Strokes for problem-solving.
- Always start with something the Stroke can achieve easily and return to it if stuck (or depressed – this advice is for both helper and Stroke!).
- Coordinate therapy sessions. If standing balance has just been achieved in the physiotherapy department, then incorporate it into occupational therapy activity; if naming objects or the use of Amer-Ind is on the agenda in speech therapy, then incorporate this into the other therapies; if the Stroke has been standing for a while in OT, then it may be better to begin with sitting activities in the ensuing session to prevent fatigue.

- Little and often is a better way to build stamina and sustain carry-over into daily activity. Even changing weight-bearing positions reinforces the natural dynamics of postural adjustments.

- Mime, gesture, repeat, rephrase, facilitate or physically prompt, and allow time for slow synapsing, if responses are unforthcoming or unexpected. If there is still confusion, analyse the cause. If stuck, go onto something else before frustration sets in.

- Monitor entire body activity and utilize mass movement synergies even during explicit limb work; it is not normal for any part of the body to work in isolation.

- Inhibit all stereotyped abnormal reflexia. Weight-bearing through proximal joints stimulates natural inhibitory systems. Normal movement generates normal movement (and vice versa). This applies **24 hours a day**, including mealtimes, speech therapy sessions, doctors' rounds and in transit between therapies in the care of a porter, except possibly in dire emergencies like earthquake, fire or cardiac arrest.

- Passive movements are not rehabilitative. If the Stroke is unconscious, limbs should be moved in large normal patterns not in their component parts, and rolling and turning should be carried out to replicate the natural movement incorporating trunk rotation.

- Static poses are unproductive; it is the control of dynamic movement that is needed to restore normal functional activity.

- Don't make a 'patient sandwich'! Work and intervene from **one** side only (the S side wherever possible), and limit physical and verbal contact to just one source to maintain concentration and avoid distraction and confusion – until distraction is deliberately introduced as a therapeutic strategy to further progress.

- Facilitate and evaluate. Be pragmatic: if it works, do it; if it doesn't, don't (try again later if it still seems potentially useful). This applies to special techniques, too. Facilitation (cueing and prompting through handling) of normal movement at all times is the primary objective. An empirical approach requires objective evaluation.

- Ensure your own CoG doesn't fall outside your own BoS. A Stroke is entitled to balance problems, but a helper isn't! Remember stability is: centre of gravity over base of support, i.e. feet apart in standing, and sit down whenever possible to utilize own body-weight and free hands for more sophisticated control (and to conserve own energy). Avoid stressing the spinal column – back problems can be irreversible.

- Make and maintain contact with specialized professionals, and seek guidance and/or cross-refer for problem-solving, or for help in recognizing problems, throughout.

Finally, always utilize familiar task-specific actions wherever possible, for maximum carry-over. Few Strokes will need to harness a horse, but for Camillo Azzopardi this was the only way he regained automatic postural control and functional use in his L arm – two years after his discharge from formal rehabilitation! Figure 10.17 shows him in action.

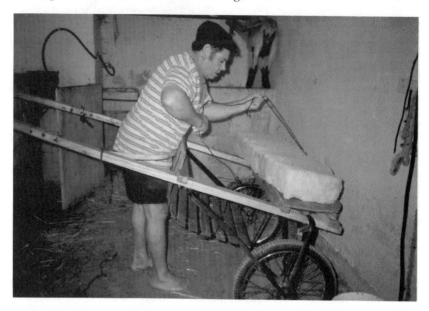

Figure 10.17 Familiar task-specific rehabilitation is the most effective: here, Camillo Azzopardi finds his own solution.

FACILITATION

Facilitation is where handling proceeds into assisted dynamic normal movements, both simple and complex. It is the basis for all skilled intervention, where unwanted abnormal patterns are inhibited and naturally recovered movement, with developing or relearned movement, is co-ordinated and manipulated into normal functional activity.

Normal movement facilitation

Support gently, but firmly, where and when necessary for movements through and against gravity, but do not give more support than is absolutely essential at any point – otherwise the Stroke will absorb only dependence on assistance from others for the manoeuvre. As recovery and relearning occurs, less physical help will be needed until certain if not all basic moves are in place again, depending on the severity of the stroke.

Anticipate and guide the initiation of component parts of the evolving sequence of moves, and the coordination of limbs and trunk, until the whole movement is completed (think of controlling the modelling of a

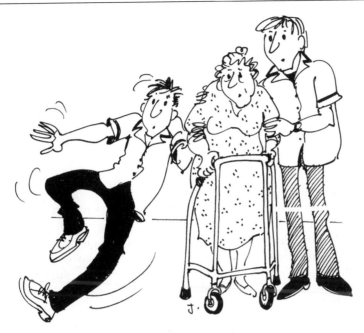

Ensure your own stability ...

wet-clay pot on a turntable). Both your hands and the judicious use of your own trunk, limbs and bodyweight can be used to support and guide the Stroke.

Anticipate and intercept to prevent unwanted moves, e.g. pressure behind the S elbow will prevent the arm collapsing into flexion if weight is to be taken through the straight arm, as in supported standing and walking, for instance.

Use pressure into musculotendinous junctions to stimulate muscle activity: this is often enough to trigger a 'stretch' response resulting in a modified contraction. For example: finger pressure into the back of the hamstrings just below the hip joint (tuck under the gluteal fold) will stimulate knee flexion for forward stepping. Follow up with verbal/gestural prompting to repeat the action consciously ('Knee up!') until the movement is incorporated naturally.

Keypoints

The automatic 'alignment', 'righting' and 'equilibrium' responses can be stimulated by the skilful manipulation of movement directed through certain points on the human form. The 'keypoints' identified by the Bobath Centre for facilitation and positive handling to elicit normal movement responses are as follows.

Central keypoint

The CoG – mid-thorax, back and front.

Threatening disturbance of CoG by applying graded pressure at the central keypoint (back or front) will facilitate automatic postural responses (including limb movement for equilibrium) in the recipient if these responses are present. Practise on friends and colleagues first to get the feel of it!

Proximal keypoints

The shoulders, pelvis (each side) and head (atlanto-occipital area and jaw). Note that facilitating from the head can be uncomfortable and feel somewhat threatening for adults.

Standing alongside or behind the recipient with a gentle but firm grasp at the shoulders, or at each side of the pelvis (whichever works best) – forward pressure will propel the recipient forwards, turning can be initiated and controlled, and gentle backward pulling stimulates stepping backwards.

Weight transference and stepping and correction of undue inward or outward rotation at the hip during walking can also be controlled. Use it to facilitate normal locomotion in the non-collapsible Stroke.

Peripheral keypoints

At the limb joints. Good rock 'n' roll dancing is the perfect example of facilitation at keypoints! The dominant partner initiates and controls the action by exerting positive pressure with the hands to partners' hips, shoulders, hands and fingers: the resulting turns, swings and spins are the normal responses (or should be, if the recipient is sufficiently receptive).

BRUSHING, TAPPING, PUSHING

Fast regular 'brushing', using fingertips (fronts or backs), over hypotonic limb musculature such as the dorsiflexors or evertors of the ankle and the extensors of the wrist and fingers, and directed upwards away from the joint in which movement is required, can stimulate a useful dorsi-flexor/extensor response. Combine with prompting as before.

'Heel strike' can be simulated to reawaken a normal but dormant response for stepping. With the Stroke sitting, gently lift the forefoot from under the toes (grasping further under the foot will trigger the PSR) until the heel is just clear of the floor and then drop the heel down again keeping the foot in dorsiflexion and the forefoot off the ground. If this triggers a reflex 'bounce' into PSR, use the other hand to maintain the

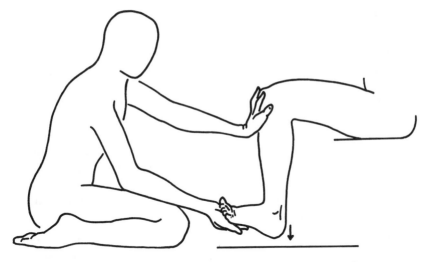

Figure 10.18 Simulating heel-strike.

S knee in flexion (downward pressure against the flexed knee) and take it more slowly (Figure 10.18). Repeat several times then replace foot carefully heel first flat on floor and start 'brushing' the dorsiflexors while prompting, 'Toes up!' Progress to assisting hip and knee flexion (one hand lifting the toes as before, the other hand grasping the shin just under the knee to push upwards) in conjunction with dorsiflexion of the ankle and toes. Progress the Stroke to standing (alongside a plinth or table – or kitchen worksurface if at home – for support if required) and bring in transference of weight for stepping, still guiding from the foot.

A similar force can be applied to the heel of the hand with the elbow extended and the arm forwards – hand-to-hand grip (as for supported walking, see Figure 10.24) and a repetitive 'pushing' action will stimulate forward push from the shoulder. Pushing against a wall is another option, incorporating elbow flexion/extension.

Never ask anyone to 'push' with the S foot (often urged when the Stroke is trying to rise from sitting to standing): it stimulates all the stereotyped reflexes, so the resulting strong extensor thrust hurls the body backwards in a twist.

10.5 PRACTICAL STRATEGIES

THE SUB-CORTICAL APPROACH

It works wonders! It prompts the use of existing 'automatic' responses, aborts undue effort, opens up networking and is also an invaluable aid to accurate assessment (like keypoint facilitation).

Always start any new activity with a sub-cortical approach. For instance:

(a) offer a bulky object, which requires two hands to hold, e.g. 'Pass me the towel', or 'Hold this for me', asked casually, and watch for comprehension, object recognition, search and location of the object, spatial awareness and flickers of spontaneous movement of S limbs, postural adjustment and bilateral limb coordination;

(b) 'Could you put your cup on the other table so that we have room to work?' adds more complexity. Element by element, it comprises: pick it up (judgement and stability – anticipating and adjusting to the added weight of both cup plus contents and arm moving away from body); turn to locate destination; reach forwards/sideways/backwards; put it down safely; regain equilibrium; and turn back to the starting position.

Indirect exercise is another way of eliciting a response. For instance, lying on the S side and moving the upper N leg to follow a moving point can stimulate supporting reactions in the S side (the same in sitting and standing).

From successfully-elicited automatic responses work towards gaining cortical (conscious) responses to specific requests for an action.

Add other movements to already-accomplished simple moves to:

- add disturbance and dynamics to a static stable posture;
- be incorporated into other activities;
- increase complexity.

BALANCE AND POSTURE

The basis for all activity. Incorporate it naturally into all activity to ensure, from the start, coordinated, controlled and fluid mass movement synergies, e.g. getting up from lying down, rising from sitting to standing and vice versa, commencing walking, turning.

Work to re-establish vertebral curves, particularly in the lumbosacral region: 'pelvic tilting' and trunk side-flexion/extension is usually replaced by a pseudo-supporting rigidity which effectively destroys vital dynamic control of posture in relation to gravity, so these movements must be regained as soon as possible.

Include in all manoeuvres, as soon as possible – once the Stroke feels confident enough not to grab at the nearest support – the onward reaching for articles (soap, walking stick, doorknob) and coping with distractions in the process.

Offering too much support encourages leaning on to or into the support. Give sufficient space to allow sway without risk, and only intervene with a supportive nudge, light fingertip pressure or verbal prompt in time to abort a total shift off balance and to ensure a gentle return to the balanced state. Have another but non-intervening helper on the N side if the Stroke veers off-balance to both sides (sitting, standing and walking), or utilize adjacent furniture/pillows/wall.

Use a pillow or two under the S elbow for sitting on the edge of the bed, or a chair arm in sitting out, or S forearm or hand supported on a table or plinth of appropriate height while standing. The pressure upwards to the shoulder will stimulate natural supporting reactions and inhibit abnormal patterning.

STANDING AND STEPPING

Involves dynamic control of the transference of body weight to govern postural sway and is the preparatory stage for walking.

The initial stages are established during sitting-to-standing routines and in transfers between bed/chair/lavatory/car etc. If these have been handled and facilitated efficiently then the natural groundwork will already be in place. If not, then work through the preparatory stages by repeating these early sequences (with variations – different height bed, chairs, chairs with and without armrests).

VARIABLE-HEIGHT PLINTHS, BEDS AND TABLES

These provide an infinite range of opportunities for rehabilitation purposes. The positions and actions refer to the Stroke in the first instance!
One variable-height (VH) plinth enables:

- Simulation and practice for getting into and out of bed, turning and rolling (on a wide plinth).
- Assisted progression to independent transfers to be practised at matching heights and between differing heights.
- Sitting balance – therapist sitting beside (with a second therapist sitting or kneeling behind if needed) until balance is achieved. With the plinth lowered a 'wobble-board' can be introduced for the Stroke to sit on for further postural activity (including the head!). Sitting with the plinth raised so that both feet are just clear of the floor enables Strokes, particularly 'pushers' and those troubled with PSR (Chapter 6), to concentrate on trunk control in sitting without reflex activity. This position can also be used with the rocking-board.
- Sitting 'hip-walking' forwards and backwards with plinth raised as above, for transference of weight (and preparatory to rising from sitting). Assistance can be given from behind to initiate and guide the pelvic rocking and rolling if needed. Once achieved, repeat with feet on floor.

- Rising from sitting and relaxing back into sitting, starting from the raised plinth with the Stroke perched on the edge, feet a little apart on floor. Starting height is relative to individual need and the plinth can be lowered as performance improves.
- Standing and weight transference in standing; facing the plinth raised to elbow height for bilateral forearm support or at a height suitable for bilateral hand/straight arm support if appropriate. This frees the therapist to work on posture and normal leg movements. Progress to stepping sideways along and around the plinth, in both directions, with synchronized moves of arm/hand. Perceptual activities and games placed on the plinth can be utilized to reinforce automatic postural control. Two or more Strokes at similar stages can participate, standing facing each other or side by side – useful for mixed therapy input.
- Standing with the S side to a raised plinth with the S forearm/elbow supported on it, stepping forwards and backwards with the N leg (with appropriate weight-transference from leg to leg between each step).
- Perch-sitting on a raised plinth, knees in slight flexion and both feet on the floor, reaching for or passing objects in all directions. This initiates and confirms coordinated supporting activity in legs and trunk.
- Sitting side-perched on the N buttock and thigh, N foot swinging clear of the floor with S leg supporting, knee bracing and S foot taking share of body weight, reaching with the N hand to various points to touch the therapist's hand or to use wall-mounted equipment. This reinforces normal supporting reactions in S leg and will stimulate and exercise hypotonic gluteal musculature (feel for it – different reaching positions stimulate different responses).

Two VH plinths are even better, particularly for working in the very early stages, from a wheelchair or with more severely handicapped (or apprehensive) Strokes, and are essential for amputee Strokes and those already disabled by other conditions, such as arthritis. One 78-year-old Stroke was admitted to hospital with a flaccid L hemiplegia, plus an above-elbow amputation of his right arm (never able to cope with a prosthesis) and a high mid-thigh amputation of his left leg (this prosthesis was unmanageable post-stroke) as a result of war injuries in 1940. He was discharged two months later, in a customized electric wheelchair with foot controls (R foot), ably independent in transfers, in and out of bed, and standing. His last few evenings on the ward he spent escaping to the local pub, standing propped against the bar (his flexible straws in top pocket ready to lip-out-and-into a glass of beer).

Do assess for, and obtain, the most advantageous bed height for each individual: too high can be as disabling as too low.

With two VH plinths:

- with the plinths a wheelchair-width apart and seat-high, and the Stroke in the wheelchair positioned facing down the 'aisle', transfers can be processed to either side – the therapist in the aisle can sit on or brace against a plinth throughout and control the action. A second therapist can work either from behind the chair, or kneeling and receiving on the other plinth.
- sitting on one plinth facing the other (a few inches away from the knees), feet flat on the floor and slightly apart:
  (a) reaching forward to place one hand (or both hands or elbows and forearms if the S shoulder-girdle musculature is relaxed and movement pain-free) on the second plinth. The BoS is extended, but bodyweight is distributed between the proximal keypoints as in quadrupeds, which initiates an upper limb supporting response in Strokes who are grabbers and pullers. Working with the N arm on a task placed on the second plinth gives dynamic weight-bearing through the S arm;
  (b) trunk flexion and the angles of movement between arm and trunk can then be increased and decreased by altering the respective heights of the plinths. This also alters the distribution of bodyweight between proximal keypoints.

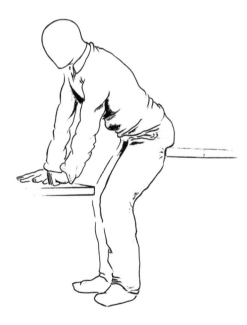

Figure 10.19 Inducing natural rising.

(c) by raising the seating plinth and lowering the second plinth to just the right levels, rising to standing and relaxing back into sitting is often automatic and irresistable (Figure 10.19): the Stroke is facilitated into re-distributing bodyweight and acquiring confidence.

Progress from this to confident rising appropriate to everyday situations by altering the levels (Figure 10.20). This can often be achieved within the same session.

If wrist dorsiflexion with fingers extended is impossible, try allowing the Stroke hand to rest 'knuckled'; arthritic Strokes can find this more comfortable with the N hand too – as long as some weight can be taken through the heel of the hand.

- if the chair is in place between the plinths, then independence in transfers to either side can be progressed easily, with education in the use of the N hand if the Stroke is elderly or obviously in need of this for ongoing use.
- with the second plinth alongside the first, kneeling can be introduced – on one plinth lowered to knee height and with hands or forearms supported on the other raised to the appropriate level to give support

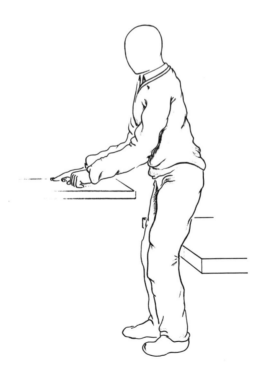

Figure 10.20 Confident rising to stand.

for comfortable four-point kneeling – progressing to just upright kneeling and balancing. This stimulates strong coordinated trunk and hip control and can be further progressed to 'walking' on the knees, forwards and backwards (less body-height to control and a larger BoS, but involving more complex synergies and 'breaking-up' abnormal reflex patterns).

- transference of weight in standing can be practised between the plinths (both at hand-support or forearm-support height). Progress to stepping and walking – forwards and backwards – incorporating normal alternate arm/leg movements.

This replaces walking between parallel bars! The difference lies in the fact that the hands/arms are on a flat surface which prevents grasping and pulling, and can readily be used as they should be – to gain alternate arm/leg swing.

A **large low (knee-high) plinth** is another really useful piece of equipment. Either super-'king'-size purpose-built with a padded top, or three singles which can be securely linked together. This allows for confident rolling and turning routines, and for early practice in kneeling and shunting towards getting on and off the floor for older Strokes prior to the actual activity (mat routines on the floor are really only suitable for younger Strokes).

It also provides an excellent relaxation bed for one or two Strokes between activities (in reflex-inhibiting positions!), and several Strokes can be grouped around the edges for specific work in sitting.

WALKING

Begins when dynamic balance is sufficiently competent in standing and stepping. In the meantime, transfer people into a wheelchair with their feet on the footplates even for short journeys – dragging someone around between two others (or singlehanded), with or without a walking frame, is not going to re-educate walking. Frequent facilitated transfers are far more therapeutic for promoting dynamic balance and recovering locomotion.

If ambition or anosognosia (or relatives or colleagues) create overwhelming pressure to start walking before this stage is achieved, then demonstrate the problem – surreptiously withdraw the total physical support that would be required, but **be ready** to control or to prevent a collapse – and allow the Stroke/relative/colleague to feel/see/assess and identify the problem for themselves.

If depression over not walking (often a misconception on the part of relatives or colleagues) is creating stress, advice and reassurance and lots more standing and stepping activities should be both beneficial and encouraging.

However, in the occasional instance it may be necessary to give almost total physical support with skilled facilitation to induce normal locomotion in Strokes who are dyspraxic, fearful or frail. In this way, normal inhibitory and excitatory systems, and normal supporting and walking patterns, may be stimulated.

Physical assistance is required to subsidize the natural supporting patterns. The helper stands alongside the Stroke to the S side giving hand support – right hand to right hand or left-to-left, helper's palm facing up palm-to-palm, thumb-to-thumb – to the almost-extended S arm held slightly forwards in relation to the trunk (Figure 10.21), with the other arm around the back to hug the opposite hip; helper's nearside hip fronting on to the back of the S hip.

Always initiate the first step with the N leg (to inhibit abnormal reflex patterning), bringing bodyweight to the S side by keeping hip contact and matching transference of weight and gait. As soon as possible encourage and facilitate a naturally alternating arm swing with each step.

Progress by judiciously withdrawing body support until the Stroke is in control, then replace physical assistance with VH plinth work.

If absolutely necessary, a second helper supports the N side in the same manner, and gait is initiated by gentle coordinated 'rocking' pressure to induce appropriate transference of weight to the S side first, preceding a step-through with the N leg. This step-through is facilitated if necessary by the step-through of the second helper's nearside leg, knee tucked into the back of the N knee. If the S knee is not bracing to take the

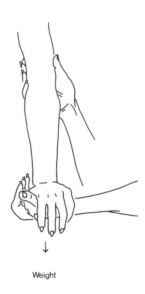

Weight

Figure 10.21 Helper's thumb-to-thumb S hand support.

transference of bodyweight, then the therapist can use his or her own offside knee pressure (from medial side of their own knee) to support the front of the S knee. Alternate this pattern to replicate locomotion, in a slightly slower than usual natural rhythm, until the first sign of participation when the degree of support can be skilfully amended – or until the participants show signs of fatigue! Progress as before.

Introduce stepping and walking backwards and sideways, sidestepping (crossing one leg in front and then behind the other), walking on carpet, over rugs, turning and manoeuvring – to open, pass through and close doors opening both inwards and outwards – around large and small objects, and jostling and distracting, and so on.

Incorporate armswing, then the carrying of articles – beanbag, handbag, bag of groceries – using N hand, S hand/arm, or both hands as relevant.

Progress to stepping over lines on the floor, over raised thresholds, up and down a single step (simulate kerbs if the real thing is unavailable), up and down stairs and include quarter turns, etc.

Finally, walk on uneven and rough ground, grass and gravel or chipping paths and, the ultimate challenge, on unstable ground such as a treadmill, bus, train or moving walkway.

Few Strokes ever regain the ability to run or jump. Both these actions require a 'push-off' from the ball of the foot which, for the S leg, triggers the PSR every time, which stops the free flow of ongoing movement dead in its tracks.

Landing with a jump – or just stepping down from a step on to the ultra-sensitive pad of the S foot – can sometimes produce the same hyper-reflexive reaction. Stepping down with the N leg each time is a safer choice for these Strokes.

STEPS AND STAIRS

A purpose-built low dais (kerb-high and portable) is useful here; it should be large enough to take a rollator with a bit of extra space around, and have a non-slip surface.

Begin with a simple step, onto the dais and then off the other side, using alternate legs. Then walk up to it and include it without breaking stride.

Walking up and down stairs should be facilitated by the helper standing a step or two below the Stroke, firming the S knee as necessary for each step and ensuring each foot is securely placed. Some hypotonic Strokes may need to take each step-up with the N leg and each step-down with the S leg in independent activities. Handrails on both sides will give reassurance to everyone! Started soon enough (before panic sets in), steps and stairs can be accepted as a normal part of everyday life after-stroke.

If coming downstairs causes undue alarm, try stepping down backwards.

If there is only one handrail, on the S side, then try facing it sideways on (carefully placed feet are even more important for these methods).

If none of this works, try sitting down and 'bumming it'.

WALKING AIDS

It is better to walk normally with help than abnormally without. Assess and make suitable provision wherever appropriate to maintain an acceptable gait between supervised therapy sessions. Strokes and well-meaning others will utilize anything available otherwise, or struggle to go it alone which may threaten or distort a newly re-acquired normality.

If it can be predicted fairly soon after the stroke that independent walking with an acceptable gait without this support is more than probable, then don't introduce a walking aid. Work directly from physical assistance to plinths to facilitation to prompting to walking unaided, but dissuade the Stroke from independent walking with unskilled help until the latter is achieved.

Strokes designated as 'mild' are often left to fend for themselves, frequently acquiring a stick in the process. Without guidance this can, in time, result in hyper-reflexia and spasticity and the traditional disabling posture of stroke due to reduced weight-bearing through the S side.

Four-legged walking frames cannot be recommended for use by any Stroke (see Chapter 8). Only Strokes with normal use of both upper limbs, good balance control and no latent hyper-reflexia should be issued with a Zimmer frame; and if they are this good they shouldn't need it (unless they used one pre-stroke: arthritics, for instance!)

For Strokes with recoverable activity in the S arm who are making slow progress in walking, the 'rollator' type of walking-frame should be used: smallish wheels on the front legs and rubber tips on the back legs which anchor the frame when weight is taken through the hands in stepping. The pushing action required to propel the frame forwards stimulates and reinforces supporting reactions in the upper limb. It also stimulates stepping and locomotion.

For Strokes who have ongoing problems with functional upper limb use, try forearm-supports fitted to the rollator. A folding three-wheeler (Figure 10.22) currently available in UK is excellent for domestic use (rear wheels are braked with hand pressure as in the conventional models).

Pushing a wheelchair while a helper controls direction and performance (and gives 'braking' resistance as necessary) is an interim option (this also assists sitting-to-rising for some people).

Tripod sticks are unstable. 'Quadrupods' (four-footed tripods!) are needed by Strokes who can manage with a walking stick but who are frail, partially-sighted, ataxic, likely to be at risk and/or living alone. It stays where it is put: it doesn't slip to the floor like an ordinary stick neces-

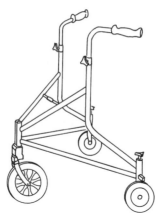

Figure 10.22 Three-wheeled, foldable, adjustable-height rollator.

sitating precarious bending and groping for retrieval. Take care that the Stroke learns to use it as a walking-stick and doesn't place it centrally to the front (this can be tripped over, and also prevents striding out) or too far to the N side as a replacement 'leg' (a ruse to avoid putting normal weight through the S leg).

Walking sticks are useful when confidence – or balance – is still a bit shaky. High enough to give a little comfort but too high to lean over on (which would reduce weight-bearing through the S side).

All walking aids need to be **adjustable** for height and adjusted for each individual.

Many elderly Strokes will have been using a stick prior to the stroke – they will still need to after it. In these cases the stick needs to be low enough to take bodyweight for the stepping-through phase.

Correct height is gauged by measuring distance between wrist-joint at base of thumb with arm relaxed by the side (not holding the stick) and the floor.

Remember: 'best foot forwards first' – it's a familiar saying, so forget the psychology – and that sending a Stroke home with a walking aid does not signify failed or inadequate rehabilitation – it indicates ongoing rehabilitation.

WHEELCHAIR MOBILITY

This should only be encouraged when active locomotion is found to be unrealistic on repeated predictive assessments. Incorporated too soon, self-propelled wheelchairing is unnecessarily effortful and because it is controlled unilaterally (by the N side) will reinforce hyper-reflexia and abnormal patterning and disrupt ongoing rehabilitation.

If a wheelchair is to be supplied, refer to experienced assessors for their advice and guidance. Interim wheelchairs for transit and transporting Strokes can be different to those recommended for independent use by the Stroke (see section 10.7).

STRAPPING, BANDAGING AND SLINGS

Accurate use can reduce oedema, inhibit abnormal patterns and stimulate hypotonic musculature.

For oedematous fingers and hands, the looser grade of elasticated control-garments (such as gloves) as used after burns can be helpful.

An ordinary arm sling should never be used. The arm position will reinforce the abnormal reflex patterns and the sling itself restricts any movement. The weight of a S arm suspended from the back of the neck is pretty unbearable, too.

To support an irretrievably flaccid arm during walking, a customized collar-and-cuff-style strap taken diagonally across the back, with arm-weight supported by the N shoulder, will prevent subluxation at the glenohumeral joint and dependent oedema/circulatory inefficiency in the hand. A single loop at one end supports the S forearm just below the elbow (held well to the front of the body), and a double loop at the other holds the S hand and fingers in midline (Figure 10.23).

If the sling slides round with activity, a push down at the S wrist with the N hand will readjust it to re-align the glenohumeral joint again.

An arm sling similar to those used to protect a traumatic shoulder dislocation can be adapted as an alternative (the band securing the arm to the chest wall isn't necessary). The 'hemi-cuff' support is featured in Chapter 8. It is ineffective. Sometimes it is sufficient for the S arm and hand to rest along the top of an over-the-head (weight on N shoulder,

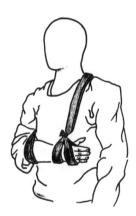

Figure 10.23 Flaccid arm support sling.

bulk under S arm) bag or satchel: the thumb web can be tucked into the front strap.

Oedematous lower limbs should respond to positioning and elastic stockings, or shaped woolly tubular pieces – in the correct size. In the short term, 'blue-line' bandaging (as for varicose ulcers) can be effective if used early enough. Straight woolly tubular bandages are not very effective unless they are tight. Shaped ones are available from the same manufacturers; they are warmer to wear, but easier to apply than the white stockings. Eradicate wrinkles in all elasticated applications and prevent them bunching up (turning rumples into tourniquets). Never turn the tops over, for the same reason.

Accurate figure-of-eight bandaging reduces ankle oedema, as do athletic ankle-supports or pressure garments if they reach to the base of the toes and the oedema does not extend up the lower leg.

In the lower limb, strapping and bandaging can also be used to facilitate normal gait. For the S knee, a couple of strips of wide elasticated sticking-plaster taken vertically to cover the spread of the quadriceps muscle bulk, from about 8 cm above the extended knee joint to the tibial insertion, and secured with a turn around the leg at the top and bottom of the strips if necessary (Figure 10.24) will not only help to stabilize the knee joint, but, as it bends, the increased sensory 'pull' on the quadriceps group gives a 'kick-start' to a 'supporting' contraction.

On hairy legs, first paint the skin with 'Tinc. Benz.' (compond benzoin tincture 'Friar's Balsam'), which makes removal less painful!

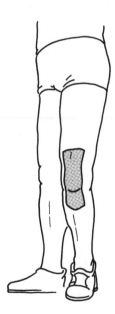

Figure 10.24 Quads-strap in place to stimulate contraction on weight-bearing.

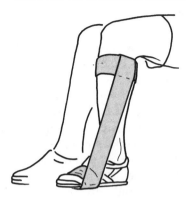

Figure 10.25 'Lively' bandaging to facilitate dorsiflexion for the S leg swing-through phase of walking.

Figure-of-eight taping with an elasticated bandage, with the S ankle in dorsiflexion and eversion, can assist heel-strike. Begin at the base of the big toe and take the bandage from the inner (medial) border under the foot first to ensure eversion.

Firm bandaging **over** the shoe prevents undue distortion in the metatarsal and metatarsal-phalangeal joints.

A stretchy bandage around the forefoot (over the shoe and from medial to lateral as before) with two or three turns to secure, and then brought taut up the outside of the leg to just below the knee and secured again with a few turns just below the knee (Figure 10.25), will often be enough to prevent the foot inverting on stepping-through while allowing a degree of natural ankle movement.

To facilitate normal stepping-through with the S leg, the bandage can be taken straight from the lateral border of the foot to be secured on to a waistband or belt above the S hip. A position slightly to the front of the hip assists forward stepping of the whole leg; one slightly behind the S hip assists knee flexion (Figure 10.26); or the end of the bandage (and its placing and tension) can be controlled by the helper alongside the Stroke.

SPLINTS, BRACES AND CALIPERS

Use with discretion!

Inflatable air-splints are used by some therapists to reduce spasticity and correct abnormal patterning. They have been found to be helpful to relax chronic spasticity for immediate use in certain cases, but unhelpful for promoting ongoing auto-inhibition.

Some hyper-reflexive S wrists benefit from a firm wrist-support to maintain midline or a slightly extended position. It has to be long enough to support the forearm up to the elbow without interfering with

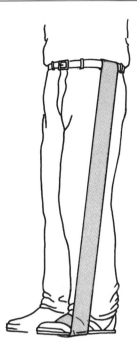

Figure 10.26 ... and to facilitate natural gait.

elbow action; if it's too short the pressure into the muscle bulk or musculotendinous junctions of the flexor groups will trigger increasing flexion of the wrist and fingers. If the fingers are already 'clawing', then a paddle-type support can be incorporated.

If ankle/foot control remains a disabling problem as independence progresses, a simple 'lively' orthosis can be applied. The one illustrated in Figure 10.27 can be used for either lower limb and fitted over any shoe with a heel of 1.5 cm or higher, otherwise the bottom coil itself will strike the ground. The spring-coiled wire with the 'lift' under the instep enables normal ankle action while controlling inversion and plantarflexion. It comes in two sizes (male and female!), the difference being in the length and the breadth. The leather ankle cuff must be firmly buckled with the lower coil tight up under the heel (Figure 10.28). Once the back strap is buckled up it needn't be undone again until the orthosis is used by someone else. Then the shin strap is fixed into place. Only the front ankle-strap and the shin-strap need to be undone for it to be taken off.

A small air-pressure splint which cradles the ankle medially and laterally, worn inside the shoe, is effective for some people.

For Strokes with really severe chronic ankle/foot inversion with plantarflexion, a more traditional spring-coiled caliper will probably need to be fitted to the shoe itself.

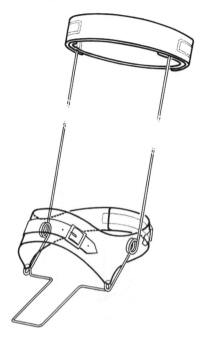

Figure 10.27 St James's 'lively' orthotic caliper.

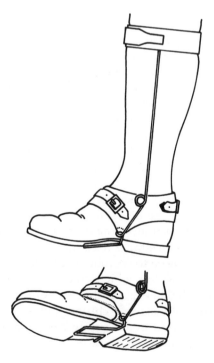

Figure 10.28 St James's caliper in place.

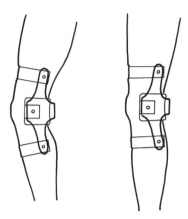

Figure 10.29 The 'Swedish knee-cage': a brace to prevent hyperextension.

Rigid ankle orthoses, customized or off-the-shelf, **do not rehabilitate normal gait** and should never be supplied. The plastic sort, worn inside the shoe, restrict movement between the small bones of the foot and cause pressure sores or callus formation at the edges, but discomfort is often unreported as most of the Strokes who seem to require them also have marked sensory loss.

Hyperextension of the S knee, on weight-bearing, is a common risk with hypotonic musculature. If walking with the knee in slight flexion is impossible, then a 'Swedish knee-cage' (Figure 10.29) will prevent the problem in the short term, until the muscles regain sufficient tone. Two adjustable straps, one above and one below the patella, hold the knee joint close into the rear bar which is mounted on the same rigid sidepieces to maintain the knee in slight flexion. Very occasionally a long-term brace may be required.

S ARM AND HAND

It is conjectured that the traditionally poor recovery of hand and arm function is due, in part, to an early lack of natural stimulation in normal weight-bearing situations. After a stroke, the lower limb is naturally used in all major body moves from turning in bed to sitting and standing, whereas the arm tends to be ignored or carried like a spare part.

It is very necessary to protect the vulnerable joints, but appropriate involvement of the upper limb in all activities – careful placing for natural direct or indirect weight-bearing to promote supporting reactions, as in getting out of bed – in addition to specific programmes including interaction and coordinated work with the N upper limb, should ensure as good a recovery as possible. For example:

- in forearm support sitting, encourage supination (turning the hand palm-up) with finger extension and thumb abduction and extension;

- the same position but with the wrist supported in midline up to the base of the fingers – or slightly 'dropped' – over the edge of a table (or book), work for active extension of the wrist and fingers;
- use a large ball (such as a toy football) for two-handed passing and collecting (facilitating S arm and hand as appropriate), and progress to full-range elbow and shoulder action for throwing and catching.

Hand and finger function require extremely complex and sophisticated networking: even a little damage will result in much greater loss of function and dexterity than is seen in the less subtle movement patterns of the lower limb. Nevertheless, persistent and careful rehabilitation should rescue much of the larger movements and in some Strokes a remarkable degree of dexterity can be recovered.

FEEDBACK AND BIOFEEDBACK

Tactile (as in facilitation), verbal and visual cues give external feedback for the re-education of normal movement. Visual cues can:

- be communicative, e.g. gesture;
- invoke gaze control, e.g. targeting a fixed or moving signal;
- be orientational, e.g. a mirror reflection of oneself, or spatially-induced, e.g. doorways, steps and so on.

Mirrors can be effective for postural symmetry, however some Strokes with cognitive impairment are unable to relate their mirror-image to their self, and a few actively dislike looking at themselves (Chapter 12).

Instant photography such as polaroid snapshots gives emphasis to postural or reflex anomalies for Strokes who cannot feel them, either as a result of proprioceptive impairment or because of neuromuscular remodelling to 'false normal'. These can also be used to demonstrate successful correction – before and after intervention – but permission must be requested from the individual concerned before any photographs are taken.

The same ethics apply to filming. Video film provides an excellent record of the rehabilitation progress. It highlights anomalies in handling and facilitation techniques as well as in individual movement and responses to stimulation. Film from all angles – beside, behind, above and below, front, quarter-front and so on. The results are educational and benefit professional practice as well as Stroke performance!

With a TV screen handy the session can be replayed immediately to the Stroke (and other interested parties with the agreement of all involved) and a workshop or discussion developed which reinforces interest and carry-over. Attention and concentration is wonderfully enhanced, too.

For many Strokes who cannot relate to mirror-imaging, watching themselves moving 'live' on screen while recording takes place is, in fact, totally meaningful (interesting, this). Leaving the equipment set up can release a therapist from continuous hands-on or verbal cueing (provided, of course, that balance and other risk factors allow this) and the Stroke will continue to work for symmetry and alignment by visual self-cueing. Again attention, concentration and carry-over are better when self-induced in this way.

Many gadgets are available which produce a range of audible or visual signals to alert the client, the therapist and the researcher to the accuracy or efficiency of the Stroke's performance to give qualitative or quantitative information. This biofeedback is discussed briefly in Chapter 11.

NEUROMUSCULAR ELECTRICAL STIMULATION

This has enormous potential and many devices are coming onto the market offering a range of modalities and protocols, from direct application to specific muscle groups to the re-laying of synergist/antagonist reciprocity, CNS plastic adaptation and trophic recoding. More detailed information is given in Chapter 11.

EXTERNAL PERTURBATION

All the strategies so far have used a fixed or pseudo-fixed base to provide the external reaction for movement against gravity – a static supporting surface (floor, plinth, chair) against which dynamic body movement can be adjusted for functional performance.

Full control of dynamic movement requires the ability to perform volitional movements even when the supporting surface itself is subjected to external perturbation. These last few strategies introduce this extra factor.

Gymnastic balls

A short formal course on the use of these is recommended; they come in several sizes and the larger versions are designed to support bodyweight and can be sat on.

Safe transfers on and off and during use must be assured: siting them between two plinths, for example, with another helper standing behind, affords an optional 'fixed base' for the actual transfer and for stability in a crisis of confidence.

Dynamic postural activity can be facilitated, and subtle automatic postural control for equilibrium is stimulated.

Moving in water

Water is a marvellous element in which to work for dynamic balance control and full use of all of the musculature involved in postural adjustment. It promotes auto-inhibition of otherwise uninhibited hypertonus, increases demand on hypotonic tissue (which provokes re-innervation) and much of the weight of otherwise 'heavy' limbs (due to ungraded muscle tonus) is taken by the water itself.

However, there are obvious risks – and certain important factors that need to be taken into account:

- first gain medical clearance from the doctor currently in possession of the medical file and facts relating to the individual Stroke.
- if continence is a problem, then immersion is inadvisable for hygienic reasons.
- ensure that the Stroke has emptied bladder and bowels prior to the start of the activity; immersion raises extra- and intra-abdominal pressure and also increases diuresis.
- a minimum of two skilled personnel per Stroke must be active participants throughout (three for two Strokes together may be acceptable for the more able); one to control from the front, one to work with the S side.
- cold triggers abnormal reflex patterns and spasticity. The water needs to be warm – hydrotherapy pools are ideal. If this is not available perhaps a local special school with a pool for handicapped children would allow access. The pool environment must be warm, too, for drying and changing.
- great care must be taken at all times in the pool environment to prevent slipping and sliding on wet floors and traumatized ankles (insecure situations produce anxiety which enhances reflexive patterning).
- poolside hoists help the getting-in and getting-out process if insufficient experienced personnel are present to facilitate and control the safe negotiation of ladder, steps or walk-in slope.
- wet skin is particularly slippery, so any grasp must be extra firm and supportive (no panic grabs at the S arm except to prevent drowning!).
- water should reach mid-sternum – lower does not give sufficient buoyancy, and effort replaces ease of movement.
- the S foot must be carefully placed flat on the floor of the pool and its position continuously supervised to ensure weight-bearing without soft-tissue injury. A helper's forefoot under the toes and forefoot of the S foot (from the lateral side) is recommended – correction can be maintained and it saves the helper continually having to duck under the surface to grapple with a slippery limb.
- fifteen minutes in the water is long enough for the first few sessions – concentration is intense, and the warmth is extremely fatiguing (all muscle tone is decreased).

- have a towel and a chair at the poolside for when the Stroke comes out of the water: their blood pressure will be lowered because of the peripheral dilation of blood vessels, and relaxation of musculature can be profound so that re-exposure to the full force of gravity can produce a sense of general weakness or extra 'heaviness' for some time afterwards.

Active exercises in the water are not needed!

At the start, the exercise is in maintaining standing balance against the random movement and pressure of the water itself, which is stirred further by the movements of the helpers who are having to maintain their own standing balance while supporting the Stroke to do likewise.

Facilitate from proximal keypoints – don't hang on to hands and arms; allow free arm movement to encourage normal equilibrium reactions.

Once the Stroke has orientated to this, introduce gentle vertical movement (both knees bend and stretch) and selective arm movement (swirling actions). The buoyancy of the water encourages freer and more controllable arm movements, and more dynamic postural adjustment is required.

Progress to the transference of weight in standing – from side to side and then in step standing, forwards and backwards – before encouraging actual stepping and walking. Continue to control the placing of the S foot and trunk symmetry.

Encourage floating: with one helper behind the Stroke, their body to the S side, with one arm under the N arm and round the front of the Stroke's chest to control anticipated rolling to the S side, the Stroke can relax back with their head comfortably nestled into the cradle offered by the helper's neck and shoulder.

With a L hemiplegia the head should go on the **helper's R shoulder**, and vice versa. This leaves the helper's other hand and arm free to support and control the S side of the pelvis to lift without twist, and to maintain own equilibrium. A second helper standing to the S side may be needed to assist with an initial lift under the hips to bring the body into a relaxed floating position.

Walking slowly backwards towing the Stroke in this way encourages relaxation and gentle participation – appropriate paddling using both feet, both hands, alternately or together. It is a pleasant way to finish a session. But proceed across the width of the pool, not the length! In one session in a hotel pool the helper walked himself backwards into the suddenly-shelved deep end and disappeared, leaving the Stroke happily floating by himself (fortunately sufficiently relaxed and unaware). The Stroke was actually overjoyed to be told of his achievement after the helper had surfaced to collect him, but the helper required a bracing whisky afterwards and still frets about the other possible consequences.

Swimming forwards is not so simple: the S arm may not be capable of such elevated reach, and unequal limb action, hyper-reflexia and reduced coordination will force the Stroke into a spiralling twist-and-turn to the S side, and downwards under the surface.

Once out of the pool, accompany the Stroke to give continued support and facilitation for showering, drying and dressing. A marked improvement is usually immediately noticeable (by the Stroke, too) and it is an ideal opportunity to progress walking and normal functional activities if the Stroke is not too tired. Carry-over of auto-inhibition of the abnormal patterns should last for an hour or more, ongoing facilitation of normal movement will extend this even further.

Other familiar perturbations which stimulate normal automatic postural adjustments include travelling as a passenger in a car, on escalators (both stairs and walkways) and horse-riding (mechanically-simulated or the genuine thing!). Camillo Azzopardi, seen in the frontispiece, has a L hemiplegia with residual raised muscle tone which makes all selective movement clumsy and awkward. Once aboard his flimsy horse-drawn trotting rig, however, he feels normal and free from this constraint. This is a nice example of the role of postural control in freeing peripheral movement and, in this situation, enabling fluent weight-transference for the unlocking effect of secondary systems of inhibition.

10.6 SPECIFIC PROBLEMS

ATAXIA

Many central or cerebellar lesions leave the Stroke with bilateral limb function (maybe reduced on one side), but difficulty in coordinating the two sides of the body.

Use the Bach-y-Rita principle (practice greatly improves but does not completely replace the lost link).

Work to increase coordination: gross movements first. Fine movements in the hands often appear unaffected but clumsy, and their usefulness will depend on synergic control of the more proximal joints.

Broaden external frame of reference (BoS) to increase the range of proprioceptive sensory stimuli, e.g. invoke upper limb support (but not from parallel bars or people!). Begin with four-point stability (both hands, both feet, firmly based).

For the upper limbs, utilize normal bilateral supporting reactions for arm movements in sitting to reinforce shoulder stability, e.g. simple 'push-ups' from the arms of a chair, or stick-work where the helper in front holds a walking stick horizontal while the Stroke, with hands on stick shoulder-width apart, pushes against resistance without leaning into the back of the chair.

Work between hip-high plinths for balance and stepping, with the plinths far enough apart to permit natural sway and transference of weight from foot to foot, but close enough to prevent overshooting, i.e. contact gives feedback. Progress to walking via alternate hand/leg stepping, ensuring three stable points of contact at any one time, i.e. moving the R hand forward, with both feet and other hand still supporting, then the L leg, then L hand, then R leg, and so on. Progress to two-point stability (moving alternate hand/leg simultaneously).

When the Stroke is competent at this, try elbow crutches – the high forearm support helps to firm up the shoulder synergies and to stabilize the hand base. Progress to walking out into a less secure environment (e.g. floorspace!).

If these seem premature, but early independent walking is a priority, introduce a rollator walking-frame.

Progress to two sticks, one stick, unsupported as appropriate. Walking between two helpers, or hanging on to one, does nothing for ataxic gait – the helpers are exercising their own dynamic balance control while the Stroke is merely learning indiscriminate pulling-on and pushing-off tactics and dependence on other-people-power and their balance-adjustment.

SYMMETRICAL TONIC NECK REFLEXES

These are often associated with a fair recovery of movement, but fully functional activity – especially rising from sitting, and walking – is compromised by the reflex patterning.

Systematically break up the patterns, first by thoughtful positioning while the Stroke works on other tasks, then proceed to dynamic postural adjustments working through the reflex patterns to functional activities and walking. Ensure that the head/neck position is posturally appropriate throughout – the Stroke may be trying to gain erect posture by the use of visual stimulation (forcing gaze upwards), which tilts the head back. This of course reinforces the reflexia.

Start with the Stroke sitting on a lowered VH plinth, leaning forward with hips and knees and elbows flexed and forearms supported on a second (higher) VH plinth, until this position is accepted. Then smoothly adjust the heights of both plinths to give:

- high perch sitting (legs almost straight) with straight arm support on lower plinth;
- facilitation to rise into standing with straight arm support;
- four-point quadrupedal stance, trunk near-horizontal, both legs and arms straight;
- repetition of sitting-standing-sitting from this position.

Work also on four-point kneeling on the plinth at knee height – if the Stroke can accept it (e.g. arthritic joints present difficulty). Progress to: high-kneeling with forearm support on the second plinth (at appropriate height); to inching forwards and backwards in this position; to repeating with straight arm support (on second plinth, appropriately lowered) with head, elbows and hips extended.

Progress to assisted walking with helper(s) ensuring straight arm support; always be prepared to facilitate elbow extension in walking. Aim for independent locomotion – walking-aids are problematic because the necessity to extend the arm(s) for support triggers the complete reflex (Figure 6.2) unless the hyper-reflexia has been successfully overcome.

If ongoing support is required after formal rehabilitation ends, try out the whole range: Zimmer, rollator, sticks, quadrupods and select the least disabling. A minority of people may need to rely on physical support for walking; arm-in-arm on the predominant S side for choice. Even with one elbow flexed, the legs will be able to function, but increasing spasticity may jeopardize this mobility in the long term.

ASYMMETRIC TONIC NECK REFLEX

As with the previous problem, functional movement is hampered or rendered useless by this reflex even where S limb activity seems to have been regained.

It is reinforced by the use of a walking stick in the N hand: as the N arm extends to take weight on the stick, the S arm will fly into flexion and the head turns uncontrollably to the N side.

Work to break up the patterns by utilizing weight-bearing at proximal keypoints.

Use visual clues to centre the head and neck during activity; stimulate and stress bilateral and symmetrical arm/hand activity.

If independent locomotion is not achieved, then advise the use of a rollator. It will reinforce bilateral supporting reactions in walking.

'PUSHERS'

Usually associated with L hemiplegia, this problem is possibly the result of:

- severe sensory impairment on the S side;
- heightened reception of tactile and proprioceptive information from the N side extinguishing input from the S side;
- unilateral neglect, which over-rides the normal bilateral protective supporting reactions in both upper and lower limbs.

The automatic equilibrium and supporting responses are therefore only initiated unilaterally, on the N side. These are the Strokes who literally push themselves over when feeling unstable in dynamic situations.

Work to stimulate and reinforce supporting reactions on the S side in both the arm and the leg (using the subcortical approach too). Progress from dynamic postural control in sitting, to standing with the S arm supporting while tasks are performed with the N hand, to facilitated conscious control.

Encourage visual scanning of supporting surfaces (including the floor!) and S limbs, to increase awareness of S limb stability and placement.

Stepping and walking can be progressed with VH plinths as for ataxia. Helper-assisted stepping and walking (facilitating S arm extension) requires a second helper on the N side to give: N hip and shoulder contact for the stepping-through phase with the S leg (but not supporting the Stroke in any way); and positive verbal reminders, 'Lean towards **me**', 'Keep hip contact', 'Stay shoulder to shoulder', to maintain bodyweight through the N leg long enough for the S leg to complete the stride. This will over-ride the tendency to 'push off' with the N leg while the S foot is still in mid-air.

Actively dissuade the Stroke from clutching, grabbing or pulling for support, as this will defeat the exercise! Independence depends on the appropriate use of bilateral automatic supporting reactions.

Progress to rollator-walking, facilitating natural supporting activity on the S side as necessary, and then (hopefully) to walking unaided. A forearm-support rollator, or a rollator (which can be adapted for one-handed use as a last resort, provided both legs are under control), or two sticks (if the S hand is functional now) may be required by those who need longterm support.

Note: given a single walking stick in the N hand, these Strokes demonstrate their bilaterally-impaired support mechanism: i.e. an inability to place the stick and use it correctly. The Stroke will not put weight through the stick but will tap it about, and wave it in the air while toppling to the left.

HYPERTONIA, HYPER-REFLEXIA AND SPASTICITY

Avoid all movement into the reflex patterns until they can be performed – and controlled – selectively. Work to reinforce movement out of the abnormal patterns.

Increase weight-bearing through the proximal joints (shoulders and hips) on the S side with careful positioning for resting between activities.

Facilitate dynamic movement using the central and/or proximal keypoints, without causing pain or increasing spasticity.

If necessary change the position slightly (or completely) until the pain has gone and abnormal tone is reduced.

General strategies

In lying:

- turning and rolling to the S side; make sure that the S shoulder isn't in a vulnerable position – scapula flat on supporting surface, for instance, and that the arm is close in to the side of the body during a complete roll;
- utilize the side-lying position for 'indirect' exercise by requesting specific movement from the N arm and leg;
- with three single low plinths fixed together (or one, purpose-built), facilitate several complete rolls in both directions (this is much more enjoyable than it sounds!); as the spasticity melts away, the S arm can be gradually brought up into elevation for ongoing rolling with both arms above the head.

Allow a rest, if necessary, in prone lying (face down) for a few minutes with the head to the N side, N arm curved up around the face and S arm relaxed down the S side (or vice versa if more comfortable), or facilitate smoothly into another activity.

In **sitting**:

- encourage the Stroke to relax forwards, head towards their knees and both arms relaxed down towards the floor each side of knees. A slow and controlled uncurling, starting from a pelvic tilt forwards, encourages normal intervertebral movement into posturally-correct upright sitting, both arms remaining relaxed by the side;
- facilitate pelvic tilting forwards and backwards, and weight-transference side-to-side.
- a skilled therapist kneeling behind the Stroke can work to re-educate normal postural muscle tone using the techniques pioneered by Mary Lynch of the Bobath Centre. These involve close hugging, with the therapist's hands and own body controlling fluid trunk movements by pressure into the central keypoint from the front and back. Do the formal course before trying it: some elderly Strokes and the big-bosomed dislike such intimate proximity (and a few just enjoy the cuddle!). Like most techniques, it works for some but not for all.
- in a wheelchair, encourage the Stroke to lean to the S side and allow the S arm to relax down towards floor (not to be confused with the forgetful dropping-off-the-armrest due to sensory impairment or unilateral neglect).

There are several techniques which impose external stimulation to limbs, such as icing (see Chapter 8) and the use of inflatable air-splints. These have not been found to be as useful in the long-term control of spasticity as those which utilize – and promote the return of – normal auto-inhibition.

Particular strategies

Hyper-reflexive flexion in the trunk and lower limbs, if unsuppressed, prevents safe sitting and any walking. It is triggered by flexion at the hip, and reinforced by sustained sitting with the hips flexed at 90° or less.

In addition to the usual strategies, work to reinforce natural extensor patterns (take care not to stimulate the abnormal extensor reflexes instead) by using positions which avoid undue hip flexion at first, e.g. perch-sitting on the edge of a raised bed or on a high stool, with the knees slightly bent and feet on the floor, heels down. This extends the hips and stimulates the supportive 'bracing' extensor responses while tasks are performed with the upper limbs. Practice lots of perching-to-standing-to-perching to reinforce this.

Once safe sitting is established in perch sitting – probably in the first session – ensure that the Stroke is given the facility to sit mostly in this position instead of in an ordinary chair, with arms supported on a **high** table (to maintain weight-bearing through the legs) for security, until the problem is overcome. Borrow a perching stool with arms and a backrest if necessary. It may look uncomfortable, but it works (in a matter of days, if adhered to).

Progress to dynamic activities involving work through, and then into and out of, hip flexion without triggering the reflexia.

Without such intervention these Strokes, and those with hyperactive extensor reactions, will join the ranks of elderly Strokes seen in long-term care, strapped into monstrous tipped-back chairs to prevent them toppling or slithering out.

These Strokes, too, often develop the flexor 'spasms' usually associated with spinal cord lesions, so that lying in bed causes the S leg to jump into flexion whenever the hips are extended (stretch reflex). Pressure sores on the heels are an obvious risk.

Hyperactive extensor reactions respond to the same technique (controlling the degree of hip flexion and extension), but in the opposite direction, i.e. low seating to flex the hips (if necessary also sitting on a wedge cushion, wide end to the front), leaning forward to lean on and work at a low table at first, and progress as before.

Electrical neuromuscular stimulation using specific protocols for spasticity (see Chapter 11), designed to reintroduce reciprocal activity and inhibition of opposing muscle groups, can be very effective with selected clients.

Injections of a paralysing toxin are still undergoing trial (although used by some medical practitioners already). The effects are short-term and long-term analysis has yet to be published.

The use of general muscle relaxants and specific anti-spasticity drugs is discussed in Chapter 11, with other forms of medical intervention.

'CHRONIC' HAND/FOOT SPASTICITY

The 'clawing' of apparently ineradicable hypertonic flexor patterning of the S hand and fingers is the result of early mismanagement and enthusiastic ball-squeezing. Hand-washing and drying is extremely difficult, which leads to fungal infections, and the nails can pierce the palmar flesh in severe cases.

Confronted with this problem, start with a few general dynamic movement activities to inhibit spasticity, then soak the hand in a bowl of warm water with the Stroke seated in a reflex-inhibiting position, leaning forwards, the bowl on a low table in front. Remove the hand before the water cools (working continuously to inhibit unwanted activity) and dry the skin carefully, separating the fingers gently one by one. Repeat for dusting with talc or an anti-bacterial powder (be guided by medical or nursing advice – specific creams may be preferred). To ease the fingers into extension and abduction, try with the wrist in full flexion to begin with. Advise everyone to repeat the process several times a day for as long as necessary, and encourage the Stroke to massage and stretch the interconnecting skin-webs while the hand is warm and relaxed, using a medicated cream or a chosen handcream. Sometimes an elasticated pressure-garment (a glove) is a useful progression.

If the chronicity of the condition does not allow a relaxed and corrected hand posture to be sustained (by interlinking fingers, for instance), try a foam 'knuckle-duster'. Snip holes through a hand-wide strip of foam to take the fingers to maintain separation; ensure a comfortable fit. Abducting the fingers **reinforces** extension at the metacarpo-phalangeal joints.

A chunky hand-wide foam wedge to hold the palm open is another option. Place the thin side into the palmar crease; the wedge must be long enough to support the finger tips without undue skin pressure. Customize it by shaping curving troughs towards the wide end to take each finger, allowing a natural open 'grasp'. It must also be wide enough to allow the thumb to curve naturally around the side. It may be necessary to support the wrist (in midline) and hand (with or without wedge) on a paddle splint.

Feet can be treated similarly, but with the bowl on the floor, and use chiropodist's toe-separators instead of the knuckle-duster or palm-wedge. Work especially to relax and stretch the medial (inner) side of the long arch under the foot, and to regain full dorsiflexion without toe-clawing.

WHEELCHAIR MOBILITY

There will be Strokes who remain unable to walk without maximum assistance, and for these people alternative means of independent or partially independent mobility must be found. In the UK there are established wheelchair clinics, and referral will ensure customized advice and possible provision. Disability Aid Centres offer a wide range for private selection and purchase. Seek professional guidance before making a decision, and helpers should try them out too, in order to be able to advise on ongoing use.

Assessment must not only match the size and type of chair to the user, and the user to the environment, but also its manoeuvrability (for the user, and within the environment): four small fat-tyred wheels are better for grass or gravel; those with two large wheels can be self-propelled (one hand, one foot if necessary) as well as pushed, and the smaller wheels can be set before or behind them.

Seat height and width should be chosen to fit each user, and for ease of transfer to other pieces of furniture, as well as its ability to pass through assorted doorways. Comfortable foot-propulsion should be taken into consideration if it is envisaged.

Optional accessories can include a tray, a folding back-support, detachable armrests, arm-support troughs and lower-leg backrests, depending on the model. Check with manufacturers.

For lengthy daytime use, special cushions will probably be necessary to protect pressure-sensitive areas.

Self-propelling wheelchairs suit a number of people for indoor use, but each individual will have different requirements. Cognitive impairments can hinder proficiency: dyspraxics may have difficulty with coordination and control; and Strokes with unilateral neglect may feel quite competent but will create mayhem to the neglected side, ranging from physical damage to themselves (scraping elbows on doorways for instance) and to others (collision), to material damage to everything else in the environment.

Single-handed control – where the N hand has to manipulate two propulsion rims (one for forwards and the other for backwards) – is complex and only a few will master it satisfactorily.

Using one hand and one foot can be very effective once the individual has found the knack of not going round in circles, but not for Strokes with residual hyper-reflexia and/or spasticity.

Set up a practice area with large and small obstacles randomly spaced, doorways, ramps and slopes amongst others. And check the brakes!

Carers will also need to gain experience in pushing – including negotiating tight turns and steps, kerbs (forwards up, backwards down) and slopes.

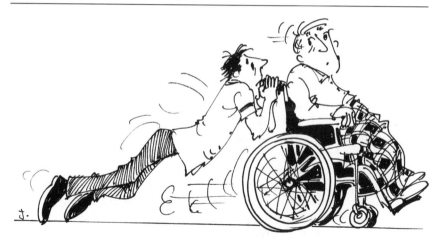

... and check the brakes!

Avoid the extended brake-lever attachment on the S side – twisting across the body to reach it with the N hand may in theory promote awareness to the S side of the body, but in practice it stimulates retraction of the S shoulder and side-flexion of the S side, which triggers and reinforces spastic hyper-reflexia, and, on returning to face forwards, the S hip will remain further back into the back of the wheelchair so that symmetrical sitting is lost. Transfers to the S side are impossible because the extended lever gets in the way; if performed regardless, the brake is likely to get knocked and released so that the wheelchair rolls backwards in mid-move. **A single brake-lever**, set on the N side, which will operate both wheel-brakes, should be requested if the S hand is not functional.

The **hand-propulsion ring** can be removed from one or both big wheels, depending on their use, in order to slim the total chair-width.

Most wheelchairs are supplied with **rubber heelstops** on the footplates to prevent feet slipping backwards and getting caught under the chair. If the user has flexor reflex patterning in the lower limb these are essential. If not, remove them to allow the feet to be placed properly and supportively with the heels further back.

The hand controls for **electric battery-operated wheelchairs** (indoor and outdoor varieties) can be set to either hand and customized also for foot or mouth control, and some can also be adjusted for separate helper control. Electric wheelchairs are heavy for loading into a car boot for trips further afield and batteries require nightly recharging from a mains supply, which may prove difficult for someone living alone.

INCONTINENCE

Introduce bladder retraining from the very beginning.

- Chart the frequency (number of times per day, and length of time between voiding) with the Stroke participating, and aim to be present in time to assist the individual to the toilet or commode. A few hectic days are worth a lifetime of misery.
- Teach pelvic-floor exercises (get advice from the physiotherapists). In the meantime, advise the Stroke to: 'Tighten all the muscles of your bottom and 'pull up' all the muscles inside. Hold for a count of five, then relax. Keep practising.' Also tell them to try to hold on a few seconds/minutes longer before emptying when you have to go to the loo', and, 'while you are peeing, try to stop the flow a few times in mid-flow'.
- Then, gradually and with mutual agreement, plan to extend the length of time between emptying. Increasing physical activity will tone up somatic musculature generally to assist interplay in abdominal pressures.
- Ensure the provision of adequate toileting – on demand, at regular intervals according to charted need – and good facilities for wiping/cleaning and hand-washing.
- Improve the environment – make it easy to reach the toilet (commode alongside, or bed/chair located near to an accessible toilet), introduce well-labelled or colour-coded toilet doors to facilitate orientation, good lighting, space to turn (and for helper), handrails, raised seat if necessary, warmth, manageable clothing, (Velcro instead of buttons or zips, wrap-around skirts or open-crotch pants, pegs to pin clothing out of the way and so on).
- Teach methods to achieve emptying – sitting leaning forwards, rocking, placing extra pressure on the lower abdomen with arms/ hands, etc.
- Avoid constipation (a full colon increases pressure on the bladder).
- Ensure adequate fluid intake. Many Strokes try to avoid drinking liquids for several valid reasons: they are afraid of choking; they are worried about urinary incontinence; or are not given the facility or assistance they require to go to the lavatory when the urge grabs them.
- Treat underlying disorders. Infection results from inefficient emptying, sitting in wet or soiled clothing and catheterization.
- Review medication. Side effects can contribute to problems with continence, and specific drugs can be prescribed to alleviate problems in certain cases.

Electrical neuromuscular stimulation using the appropriate protocol can re-innervate denervated muscle tissue in certain cases, and re-educate it in some others (further information on this and medication is given in

Chapter 11). In a project to reduce lower limb spasticity in paraplegia by using reciprocal activation of the agonist and antagonist muscles of the thigh, Shindo and Jones (1985) noted that in 16 out of the 31 patients studied effective bladder capacity increased to allow 'dry' periods, and problems of constipation decreased in 14 cases.

If, in rare cases, urinary continence remains irrecoverable, condom- type non-invasive catheterization is an option for males. For females, and if non-invasive equipment is impracticable for males, invasive catheterization is the last resort. Intermittent catheterization to clear residual urine may be an option – in which case intermittent self-catheterization can be taught (depending on the individual) or the carer can be taught to do this.

Faecal incontinence

Approximately 1 in 200 adults in the general population suffer from regular faecal incontinence; the most common cause is faecal impaction from chronic constipation. Avoid constipation by ensuring that the Stroke has an adequate diet (plenty of fibre), and by increasing fluid intake.

If faecal impaction has occurred, then intervention is essential: clearance by repeated enemas or manual evacuation, followed by measures to prevent recurrence.

Other causes are severe diarrhoea, damage to the pelvic floor requiring medical or surgical intervention and neurogenic disorders.

Increasing physical activity and good diet (and possibly electrical neuromuscular stimulation) may be sufficient to restore natural function.

Surgery to restore the ano-rectal angle may be an option, and a permanent colostomy may be preferable to the personal and social restrictions imposed by intractable faecal incontinence.

CHEWING AND SWALLOWING

Lip closure, tongue action and coordination of the phases of swallowing are vitally interlinked. Many deaths are attributable to careless or unsupervised feeding, resulting in:

- the aspiration of liquid or solid matter into the lungs, producing a fatal pneumonia;
- choking and asphyxiation.

Any Stroke with dysarthria and all those with dysphagia must be referred urgently to a speech and language therapist (the only professionals specializing in feeding and swallowing problems) and guidance requested for ongoing management. In severe cases it may be necessary to introduce a nasogastric tube for controlled nutrition in the early stages; this is a medical procedure.

Textures of liquids and solids play a significant part in the success or failure of any oral feeding. Hot liquids, crumbly biscuits and dry mince are difficult for these Strokes to control and therefore dangerous, as are mixed substances like cereal with milk, sloppy mince and soup with bits in. Ask the experts for advice with each individual case.

In the meantime, bear in mind that:

- feeding-mugs with little spouts should **never** be used, except when swallowing is normal but the hands are too shaky to hold a cup without spillage. With a spout to the lips, the head has to tilt backwards for the liquid to pass through, which means it can jet straight down into an unguarded airway.
- thick gluey consistencies, such as porridge, are easier to manage. Dieticians can recommend thickening agents for drinks and suitably gungey but nutritious proprietary drinks and foods.
- things that really need biting and chewing, such as a simple sandwich (but not containing loose bits like egg or grated cheese), can stimulate the normal swallowing sequence.

Techniques for assisting feeding in these cases should be added to the list of common core skills for that particular Stroke. A detailed description is given in Part Four.

Licking lollipops and sucking ice-lollies on sticks (or small ice cubes contained in sterile gauze or muslin) controlled by the helper will stimulate tongue movement and reduce tongue spasticity. Nourishing drinks, including coffee, can be frozen and enjoyed this way.

Teach exercises for the facial and oral musculature, and encourage practising with the help of a small hand-mirror: tongue placing inside and outside the mouth; exaggerated mouthing of the five vowel sounds (a, e, i, o, u) for the lips; blowing-out the cheeks with the lips compressed; nose wrinkling-up; eyes squeezed-shut and opened wide; eyebrows up and down; the lot.

Tiny-movement circular massage with the fingertips to the facial muscles will stimulate circulation and tone and active movement. Make sure the action is up and into midline (nose) to avoid dragging the tissues further downwards.

Sucking and blowing exercises help to strengthen oral musculature (including the soft palate) and to coordinate respiratory control. Use wide plastic tubing, then progress to drinking straws, but not for sucking in liquids until swallowing is achieved. Blowing through a straw into liquids to create bubbles is therapeutic, though!

Breathing exercises, 'huffing' (forced expiration) and assisted coughing, taught by the physiotherapists, should also be practised.

SPEECH AND LANGUAGE

Request advice from the speech and language therapist for appropriate strategies to use with each individual Stroke. Ensure a quiet and undistracting environment while working, and don't force the pace. As with movement, effort and stress exacerbate the problems.

Be optimistic about future recovery in conversation with both the client and their relatives (see Chapter 12): verbal and non-verbal communication will continue to improve given the right encouragement, and there are no time limits. Speech therapists specializing in language problems following head injury have suggested that recovery and relearning in this area improves after the other systems have stabilized in rehabilitation, when concentration can be better channelled.

Use simple gestural communication – such as Amer-Ind – routinely, and encourage everyone else to do so (some Amer-Ind signs are illustrated in Part Four). If the Stroke finds learning a formal gestural language difficult, work to develop a personalized gestural vocabulary utilizing the Stroke's own interpretive repertoire. Allow plenty of time for word-finding and hesitancy.

Prompt articulatory dyspraxics by drawing attention to their own mouth and – with slight exaggeration – slowly form the start of the word with own lips/tongue.

Deflect perseveration – mimicking or repeating the perseverated words back to the Stroke compounds the problem. Hearers need to interrupt and prompt the correct word or introduce another word in order to open access to the Stroke's lexicon. Or change the subject.

There are a variety of devices on the market for the speech-impaired – from hand-held keyboard printouts to computerized panels which offer a selection of phrases or replicate speech. These demand appropriate skills and only a few Strokes will find them useful. The speech and language therapists will advise on the need and suitability.

Public reaction to disabled speech depends upon the degree of understanding of the cause and effect. Rehabilitation includes explanations which should travel ahead of the Stroke's re-entry into the community.

The Stroke Association (in the UK) sells plastic 'credit cards' which many dysphasic people find useful to carry. One side takes the Stroke's name, address and telephone number, the other reads:

> I HAVE HAD A STROKE
> and find it difficult to SPEAK, READ or WRITE
> I usually understand what is said
> but it helps if you speak clearly
> Your help and patience would be
> appreciated. THANK YOU

MEMORY

Memory is a complex process which is unlikely to respond as a 'mental muscle' (Sunderland *et al.*, 1983), and current evidence does not support attempts to retrain memory processes (Moffat, 1984). There is no evidence that memory can be rehabilitated; repetitive tasks that re-lay lost or impaired motor skills do not improve memory. Therefore it is necessary to utilize learning or relearning ability and to develop strategies that circumvent the problem:

- Mnemonics, first letter prompting, or picture diagrams and association. The author's name, 'Polly', is successfully remembered by several memory-impaired Strokes who learned to visualize and associate it with a parrot perhaps, or with putting the kettle on. (One Stroke can only conjure up 'Porky', but perhaps this too is picture-associated!)
- Mental retracing – returning to the original encoding, e.g. when setting off to fetch something but forgetting what it is on arrival, return (physically if necessary) to the starting point where the original stimulation (usually visual) will clue recall.

So, introduce support and self-help strategies. Teach the Stroke to use existing skills more efficiently. Work on prospective memory to replace retrospective memory, ie. learn or relearn. Colour-code doors, locate and identify high-visibility structures at strategic points for reorientation, and so on.

DYSPRAXIAS

Ideational dyspraxias are unable to carry out sequential acts automatically or to command, therefore verbal directions (and 'conductive education[1], which uses repetitive verbalization with every movement component – 'I bend my elbow') are useless.

Increase all sensory cueing, facilitate, practise and search for better strategies and more effective methods.

Ideomotor dyspraxia requires subcortical stimulation and all the facilitation strategies, and familiar and task-specific programmes, e.g. repetitive action-specific cueing in everyday activities, such as facilitating transfers between chairs again and again, talking it through until the Stroke can repeat the activity in response to visual or verbal indicators only. Some Strokes succeed by talking themselves through the sequences (a modified form of conductive education, but endorsing task-specific sequential moves, not the component parts of each movement). David, featured in Chapter 7, did this, learning to mutter his way independently through life: 'Hold banister, step down with left leg...', which is why he froze when his wife distracted his train of thought.

OTHER COGNITIVE IMPAIRMENTS

Recent literature (Wood and Fussey, 1990) suggests that rehabilitation of brain-damaged individuals should take a broader perspective, away from merely testing performance in pre-set artificial tasks and towards addressing the motor, language and memory skills displayed in every-day activities. It still recommends the training of basic cognitive skills, but now proposes utilizing these skills in the context of social and functional familiar behaviour. This endorses the newer thinking of the other rehabilitation professions, but, with the encouragement to expand conceptual horizons, psychologists are advised that 'theory should be scientifically based and capable of formal scientific evaluation' (Wood and Fussey, 1990). For therapists this creates something of a Catch-22 situation, given the subject matter. How scientific can a base be when so much that is 'known' about the central nervous system is still in fact conjectural? However, and in the meantime, work to gain and maintain attention to the task in progress and utilize all the sensory clues (visual, tactile, proprioceptive, verbal, auditory etc.) needed to initiate, sustain and complete an activity.

For Strokes with **shortened attention-span** (poor concentration), find something that will interest the individual. Start with very short simple tasks (finding a particular page of objects related to a known hobby in an illustrated catalogue, for instance) and gradually add components to maintain interest and extend the attentional time required. Widen the range to include other people's interests too. A stroke tends to isolate the individual very quickly into total self-absorption, initially for coping and then from habit (or a perceptual deficit such as anosognosia).

For **unilateral neglect** work to reinforce attention and action to the S side in every activity and at all times, 24 hours a day if possible. Accurate positioning of body, limbs, furniture and other people, to stimulate spatial awareness to the neglected side, is of the utmost importance from the very beginning for Strokes with this extra-disabling problem.

Initiate eye contact from the centre front and re-educate scanning to the S side using bold, bright or highlighted objects to indicate static and moving visual parameters. The problem is modified by effective rehabilitation, and as physical recovery proceeds and movement on the S side is coordinated into bilateral activity.

Anomalies in **spatial judgement** are not due to defective eyesight or dementia. This is a cognitive dysfunction and as such can affect independence if unrecognized and unresolved.

Casebook example

A young woman, in desperation, turned up in a taxi at the local stroke unit accompanied by her mother. Her distress, compounded by some speech and language problems, needed immediate investigation. She was discovered to have been housebound – in fact on most days she was unable to walk about or to go up and down the stairs – since her stroke six months before, despite having made a relatively good physical recovery (diagnosed a 'mild' stroke by the GP, and therefore not referred for any further assessment or therapy).

She was found to be unable to differentiate between two- and three-dimensional outlines. For example, trotting up and down stairs was fine, if she didn't look at them. If she did, then the lines of the treads registered as two-dimensional straight lines as though flat on the floor. Having fallen badly several times, she was now too afraid to attempt them. After this she found herself fearful of every movement indoors: the edges of rugs and mats became new obstacles; thresholds and doorways (with lines between different carpets, rooms and so on) loomed ominously. Everyday life was a nightmare of hesitation, guesswork and decision-taking, shuffling, falling, groping and sometimes even crawling on hands and knees. Outdoors became equally frightening: kerbs were indistinguishable from lines on the pavement and road markings, double-line road markings could be steps, and zebra crossings could be a flight of steps (up or down, no clues), and she fell or tripped continuously even when escorted arm-in-arm.

Her teenage children and her husband had become impatient and neglectful, complaining about 'neurotic' and 'attention-seeking' behaviour. Referral to a psychiatrist had not cured it; a suicide attempt brought treatment for severe depression as well as for behavioural problems.

For this Stroke, a simple walking stick provided some solution. It could be used discreetly to tap and sweep ahead of the feet to locate and define flat surfaces, steps upward or downward, and, if a step, the height or depth could be judged against the stick. Slowly returning confidence, familiarity with her environment and trying 'not to look' enabled her to move around indoors and for short local trips in the neighbourhood. Places further afield and shopping precincts still required an arm-in-arm escort, mostly for reassurance; presented with a logical explanation her friends undertook responsibility for her social life. It was too late to save her marriage and her relationship with one of her children, though, but she was gutsy and still coping a year later.

Teach the cognitively-impaired to look, listen and feel – to be receptive to clues and cues – to recognize and utilize all the intact sensory pathways to supplement and compensate for the lost or damaged perceptions.

10.7 PREDICTIVE ASSESSMENT

Stimulation (visual, auditory, tactile and proprioceptive) normally invokes a relevant response. Following a stroke, it is these responses – elicited in formal and informal situations – which are assessed and analyzed to give the baseline for any intervention (cortical and sub-cortical stimulation and indirect exercise, section 10.5). Work system-atically through the sensory list.

Visual responses include:

- getting and maintaining eye contact for stationary and moving targets;
- adjustment or realignment of posture to gesture and to mirror-imaging or reflection;
- movement to gestured instructions.

Auditory responses encompass:

- movement to spoken simple instructions;
- movement to spoken but more complex instructions;
- dysphasic Strokes obviously require non-spoken cues as well.

If volitional responses are not forthcoming, test again for an automatic response. If responses are poor or lacking in any one category, go on to augmenting one set of clues with another, e.g. visual and verbal clues together (gesture while speaking), or tactile and visual (gesture and physical prompt).

The results indicate the extent and severity of post-stroke problem areas and highlight those problems requiring specific intervention by specialist professionals.

With experience it is possible to add tasks or to demonstrate strategies to each test at each stage in such a way that the assessment not only becomes part of the rehabilitation process for the Stroke, but also gives the assessor sufficient information towards predicting outcome.

The (very) simplistic guide to predicting possible outcome in terms of dependency shown in Table 10.1 was devised for use in stroke rehabilitation. It was developed during a two-year survey into length of stay on a stroke rehabilitation unit, and depends upon a good understanding of normal human motor and cognitive behaviour and consequent impairment due to a stroke. Responses to stimulation are assessed and clumped into three basic categories, and these indicate very broadly the presence and influence of cognitive anomalies, which in turn gives an indication of the implications for long-term planning.

Table 10.1 Guide to predictive assessment for long-term planning

Responses	Processing	Eventual outcome
Accurate Volitional	Unimpaired	Probable functional independence even with limb 'loss', relative to pre-stroke status. Could live alone?
Automatic only	Impaired	Reduced independence even with full movement. Will need a minder?
Disordered Chaotic	Dysfunctional	Dependence even with full movement.

TO SUMMARIZE

Observe, feel, question, listen and explain; test, assess, analyze, evaluate and apply clinical reasoning; repeat *ad infinitum* and **learn**. These are the basic ground rules for **all** problem-solving strategies.

In nature there are neither rewards nor punishments – there are consequences.

(*Robert Ingersoll*)

REFERENCES

Fenton, J. (1989) Some food for thought. *Health Service Journal*, 666–7.

Kidd, G.L. (1992) Physiotherapy, syntax and semantics. *Physiotherapy*, **78**(5), 344–8.

Moffat, N.J. (1984) Strategies of memory therapy, in *Clinical Management of Memory Problems*, (eds B. Wilson and N. Moffat), Croom Helm, London, pp. 63–89.

Sarton, M. (1988) *After the Stroke*, The Women's Press, London.

Shindo, N. and Jones, R. (1987) Reciprocal patterned electrical stimulation of the lower limbs in severe spasticity. *Physiotherapy*, **73**(10), 579–82.

Sunderland, A., Harris, J. and Baddeley, A.D. (1983) Do laboratory tests predict everyday memory? A neuropsychological study. *Journal of Verbal Learning and Verbal Behaviour*, **22**, 341–57.

Wood, R.Ll. and Fussey, I. (1990) Towards a model of cognitive rehabilitation, in *Cognitive Rehabilitation in Perspective*, (eds R.Ll. Wood and I. Fussey), Taylor & Francis, London, pp. 3–25.

OTHER SOURCE MATERIAL

Sackley, C.M., Baguley, B.I., Gent, S. and Hodgson, P. (1992) The use of a balance performance monitor in the treatment of weight-bearing and weight-transference problems after stroke. *Physiotherapy*, **78**(12), 907–13.

Medical intervention, medication and modern technology

11

In the field of observation, chance favours only the prepared minds.

(Louis Pasteur)

Everything has to start somewhere, and diagnosis is a good start for rehabilitation. It involves investigations to eliminate stroke-mimicking pathologies and formal identification leads, more often than not, to professional intervention and treatment. Which is where modern technology comes in.

However, a large and growing number of 'Strokes' are not referred for investigation, nor admitted into a hospital bed. Instead they may be referred directly for rehabilitation. The physical handling and facilitation of normal movement can, and in many instances does, actually precede and contribute to a formal diagnosis, and medical intervention can be subsequent to changes occurring or discovered during – or as a result of – the rehabilitation process.

That is why this chapter is here, towards the end of the book:

11.1 Diagnosis
11.2 Medical intervention
11.3 Surgical intervention
11.4 Medication
11.5 Modern technology

11.1 DIAGNOSIS

Fast and accurate diagnosis of stroke is essential, but not always possible. The whole range of diagnostic tests should be available in an ideal health-care system to ensure that all apparent Strokes can be effectively screened and appropriate treatment initiated. Despite tremendous advances in diagnostic technology, however, much of the high-tech equipment required, together with its experienced personnel, is still unavailable for use in many areas. Diagnostic errors are therefore common. It has been suggested that up to 15% of patients are falsely diagnosed as suffering from a stroke. Numbers are not available of those wrongly diagnosed as not having suffered from a stroke! Many of these victims are probably perceptually rather than physically impaired, and will form part of the psychology and psychiatry caseloads. Others suffer from the popular myth that recovery from a 'mild' stroke is complete, so that latent residual problems tend to be divorced from the original event.

Casebook example

One little lad aged 14 had a stroke which the paediatricians did finally diagnose, but, because he quickly regained full limb movement, he was discharged without a referral to the rehabilitation team. Six years later his family doctor sent him to a physiotherapist for assessment. In the meantime he had experienced misery at school: poor at sports because he was uncoordinated (increased muscle tone plus some dyspraxia), and referred to educational psychologists for 'Hysterical paralysis'.

Aged 20 and with excellent exam results, he had difficulty finding work (he looked 'spastic') and was now struggling to keep a job in the parts department of his local garage ('Doesn't move fast enough'). In fact, by this time he was virtually crippled by hyper-reflexia and the chronic spasticity resulting from years of struggling to keep up with his peer group.

Given accurate diagnosis, preventive measures can be undertaken to reduce both the scale of acute damage and the occurrence of further incidents. Although certain conditions are common to all age groups, it is important to remember that just as the incidence of stroke increases with advancing age, so do a number of other disorders which may cause diagnostic confusion. Intercurrent illness or a previously unrecognized stroke can also obscure the facts.

Differential diagnoses include:

- intracranial or spinal space-occupying lesions such as tumour and abscess;
- post-traumatic encephalopathy;
- labyrinthine vertigo;
- migraine;
- meningitis;
- epilepsy;
- vertebrobasilar occlusion in cervical spondylosis ('drop attacks');
- senile dementia;
- coronary occlusion;

- meningovascular syphylis;
- convulsive disorders, such as Todd's palsy;
- neurological conditions, such as multiple sclerosis and Parkinson's disease;
- baro-receptor hyper-reflexia.

Some 'purists' also exclude strokes caused by: ruptured berry aneurysm; subdural haematoma; and other haemorrhagic lesions. However, the effects are indistinguishable from those caused by embolism or thrombosis – apart from the likelihood of more severe focal and local destruction – so rehabilitation follows the same lines and makes the same assumptions.

Predisposing (to stroke) conditions include:

- polycythaemia (excess of erythrocytes);
- hypoglycaemia or diabetes;
- sudden cardiac arrhythmias;
- Stokes–Adams attacks;
- metabolic disorders;
- cranial or extracranial arteritis;
- congenital abnormalities in arterial structure (often familial);
- cardiovascular disease risk factors;
- high blood pressure;
- atherosclerosis;

and any acute pathological incidents creating emboli such as myocardial infarction or surgery.

Diagnostic procedures include:

CAT/CT scanning (Computerized Axial Tomography). This involves sending a narrow X-ray beam through the head and measuring the amount of radiation that gets through. Measurements are made at hundreds of thousands of different orientations (axes) and fed into a computer to produce a cross-sectional picture (at any level and angle required) that can be photographed or displayed on a TV monitor.

Figure 11.1 shows a transverse slice through the level of the pineal gland (bright white due to calcium in the gland) and the anterior horns of the lateral ventricles, scanned 44 days post-stroke. According to the medical notes, the 52 year-old Stroke concerned had 'developed an abrupt onset of dysphasia and right-sided weakness, and subsequently made a good recovery'.

Timing is crucial to most of these techniques: too early and actual loss is not resolved (30–50% strokes scanned show no abnormality in the acute stage); too late and it may **be** too late. CT has been called the 'haemorrhagic excludergram' – if a bleed is indicated, then surgical intervention will probably be required urgently, if not then anti-coagulant/anti-embolytic intervention can be started.

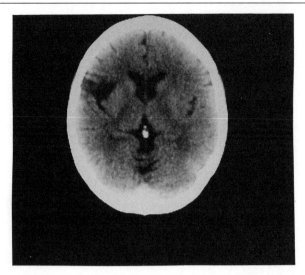

Figure 11.1 CAT scan: cerebral infarct, frontal region of L hemisphere. (By courtesy of Dr A. Colchester, Guy's Hospital, London.)

MRI (Magnetic Resonance Imaging) uses strong magnetic fields, radio-frequency pulses and computers to compose the image, which is produced by variations in the energy level of hydrogen atom nuclei in the body in response to the radio-frequency pulses. It gives a much more precise picture of the area than the CT scanner because it does not use X-rays and therefore 'sees' through bone to clearly define soft tissue structure.

Figure 11.2 shows a transfer MRI close to the top of the lateral ventricles soon after the stroke, and shows a well-demarcated zone of high signal in the R occipital and parietal region due to an infarct. The patient 'experienced a sudden onset of left-sided weakness and left homonymous hemianopia'.

Some 20% of the population cannot be screened: those with pace-makers or other internal metallic objects, such as hip prostheses, for instance.

Investigations to confirm a diagnosis of stroke include:

- CT scan;
- MRI;
- Blood count for anaemia, polycythaemia;
- Blood sugar, urea, electrolytes;
- ECG: an electrocardiograph traces cardiac rhythms;
- CSF: cerebrospinal fluid taken via lumbar puncture indicates the presence of blood and/or infection;
- US: ultrasound scanning – transcranial Doppler sonography – can detect arteritis, for example;
- Angiography: a dye which shows up on X-ray is injected into the circulatory system to define blood flow. If a blockage or partial

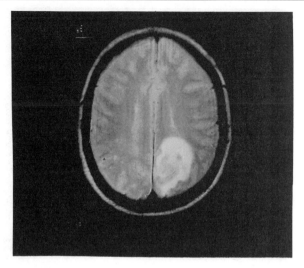

Figure 11.2 MRI: infarct in the R occipital/parietal region. (By courtesy of Dr A. Colchester, Guy's Hospital, London.)

blockage of a vessel is seen, then surgical intervention may be indicated (endarterectomy, for instance). Angiography is only an option when the risk of further stroke is under 1%, as the procedure itself involves risk (more atheromatous plaques or emboli can be detached into the blood stream).

11.2 MEDICAL INTERVENTION

Early (within eight hours of onset) treatment to reduce cytotoxic oedema and thereby minimize damage is still controversial. The use of steroids, glycerol etc. features in many trials, but so far without conclusive evidence either way. One unconvinced researcher suggests that it merely raises the severe-stroke-survivor up a category, from 'dead' to 'I wish I was dead'. However, casebook studies do seem to indicate that later judicious use of a steroid such as dexamethasone can be beneficial in selected individuals where delayed arousal or recovery is giving cause for concern.

Raised blood pressure immediately post-stroke is not significant. On-going high blood pressure needs investigation and, probably, treatment.

Airways need to be maintained. Intubation and/or ventilation may be necessary to maintain adequate respiration.

Insertion of a **nasogastric tube** for feeding ensures hydration and nutrition when the swallowing mechanism is impaired. Speech and language therapists will advise on the length of time that it is required for and how to re-introduce oral feeding. Videofluoroscopy (X-ray screening of swallowing activity using a high-definition substance such as barium) indicates the degree and extent of impairment. The technique is something of a Catch-22 and hazardous as swallowing is known to be already impaired. An experienced speech and language therapist should be present to advise and facilitate the accurate sequencing, and to try and prevent aspiration of the liquid into the airways – but this minimizes the impairment, except to expert interpreters – with suction apparatus and emergency intervention on stand-by.

Treatments designed to reduce clotting by lowering the progression of platelet adhesion embolism are clearly potentially hazardous if undertaken without certain knowledge of the nature of the vascular event causing the stroke: enhancing blood flow in haemorrhagic strokes could be fatal.

Low dose anticoagulants such as heparin are used to prevent further embolic or thrombotic strokes when these are the known cause. An aspirin a day is another simple option in these cases.

Vasodilators can lead to blood-steal situations and lowered blood pressure.

Venesection (the alternative to leeching!) may be required for polycythaemia when the corrected red-cell packed volume is higher than 48–50%.

Catheterization has already been discussed (Chapter 10). Do try to dissuade doctors/nurses from taking this step until all the conservative measures have been given time to succeed. Too soon and any recovery of continence is jeopardized; it also causes urinary infections which further delay recovery. **It really is a last resort**.

11.3 SURGICAL INTERVENTION

Neurosurgery is urgently indicated in deteriorating haemorrhagic strokes or to prevent incipient disaster from an enlarging aneurysm. Procedures include clipping off the leak or the bulge, resection and suctioning out pooled blood or haematoma. These patients are often more severely handicapped due to the extended area of brain damage incurred as a result.

Surgical treatment of **thalamic pain** falls into two groups: destructive procedures and neurostimulation.

Destructive procedures include:

- Cordotomy. If the symptoms do not affect the head or neck, cervical or upper thoracic cordotomy with division of the spino-thalamic tracts may improve the symptoms. This can be performed either percutaneously, utilizing radiofrequency thermocoagulation, or as an open procedure (Gildenberg, 1984).
- DREZ lesion (multiple lesioning of the dorsal root entry zone) may alleviate localized symptoms from the body (Young, 1990; Sampson and Nashold, 1992).

- In neurostimulation a series of electrodes are positioned – either by open surgery or percutaneously, in close relation to the CNS – which can then be driven by some form of pulse generator. This produces a tingling in the region of the pain which masks the pain itself and may give impressive, even total, pain relief. The precise mechanism of the action is unclear; whether this is a general stimulation of proximal spino-thalamic fibres or local inhibition has yet to be determined. However, clinical efficacy has been proven over the years in a number of cases (Rawlings *et al.*, 1992).

The electrodes may be positioned in either the spinal epidural space (Simpson, 1991) or deep within the brain, and these are connected via a subcutaneous lead to the pulse generator. This resembles a cardiac pacemaker and may contain its own power supply or be driven externally via an induction coil.

If direct thalamic stimulation is desired, the electrode is positioned stereotactically, usually in the nucleus ventralis-lateralis of the contralateral thalamus. Current electrodes are combinations of four electrodes on a single lead which can be programmed externally by a lap-top computer, allowing a degree of flexibility in the actual area of stimulation to best suit the individual symptoms.

Spinal electrodes similarly incorporate four electrodes, which again allows optimum positioning of the evoked responses (the 'tingling') by selecting combinations of anode and cathode.

Cardiac and vascular surgery could include: the fitting of a cardiac pacemaker; carotid endarterectomy; reconstructive surgery of a carotid artery; and extra/intracranial arterial anastomosis to prevent TIA.

Orthopaedic surgery in later stages is usually to repair acquired trauma such as fractured bones, ruptured tendons and ligaments. Rehabilitation for these procedures should accommodate the stroke rehabilitation programme too.

Occasionally it may be considered necessary to surgically lengthen or sever (release) chronically contracted and shortened tendons which hinder mobility. As these are the product of severe spasticity (if developed post-stroke), the usefulness of such a procedure should be thoroughly explored with the multidisciplinary team first. Expected post-operative improvement in position or movement in these cases is jeopardized by the continuance of the original reflexive stereotyped patterns which will then compromise other tissues.

Casebook example

A 'mild' Stroke who was never referred for rehabilitation or advice was sent for surgery after several years to have the extensor hallucis longus tendon (to the big toe) severed on the S foot. He had presented with spastic clawed toes, and the big toe was rigidly upright (possibly due to a rampant PSR). One year later he was discovered in great pain and hardly able to walk. The toe had been twisted into medial rotation by the other tendons acting on it (lose one 'tethering-rope' and the toe is subjected to the remaining forces) so bodyweight was being taken through a disturbed joint and the side of the toe, and the edge of the toenail was being driven deep into the flesh. Previously hemiplegic gait had been rendered even more abnormal through the induced imbalance and further distorted by trauma and the consequent pain. Possibly amputation of the toe could be considered next, but the underlying cause is still present with the potential to disturb and subvert any future course of action.

Alternative conservative measures could include serial splinting (to grow more sarcomeres, Chapter 3) and working to inhibit hyper-reflexia: spastic reflex patterns are often mistakenly diagnosed as 'chronically contracted' tissue. Sometimes they are – in really longstanding bed-ridden or neglected chairbound cases – but more often they are not.

Procedures to shorten the tendons of denervated muscle may be mechanically effective in some cases: a grossly subluxed glenohumeral joint due to irretrievably flaccid non-supporting musculature could be hitched up with a surgical tuck in the lax tendons, for instance. As with underlying hyper-reflexia and acquired hypertonia, the hypotonicity is likely to affect the whole muscle group and therefore the potential outcome needs to be assessed prior to intervention.

Surgery for incontinence: post-anal repair can restore the ano-rectal angle in selected cases, where faecal incontinence results from low muscle tone or flaccidity. Very rarely – usually for younger Strokes – a colostomy is performed when continence is irrecoverable and quality of life is deemed to be severely threatened.

It is now possible to form a **urinary continence stoma** – do investigate the chances of having this performed, even in older Strokes, instead of permanent catheterization for long-term urinary incontinence.

11.4 MEDICATION

This section briefly surveys some of the prescribed drugs associated with stroke rehabilitation. Doctors prescribe, but are sometimes unaware of the range of preparations applicable to rehabilitation, and also may not be familiar with the particular effects that many products have on an already damaged CNS. Discussion is always valuable, and do involve the pharmacists themselves wherever possible – they are the experts on the subject.

Up-to-date copies of prescribing guides such as *MIMS* (Monthly Index of Medical Specialities) and the *BNF* (British National Formulary) in the UK, and over-the-counter publications such as *Medicines*, give abbreviated details of proprietary preparations with brand and generic labels. Use a recognized reference and keep looking for new information – this is a complex and active field!

As with all medication there will be side effects, contra-indications and interaction with already prescribed drugs – so prioritizing is essential. Elderly people are particularly susceptible to drugs, especially to those which affect the CNS, and many are already on a regime for other disorders. In general, prescriptions for the acquired problems of stroke should be regarded as a short-term measure, to control excessive difficulties long enough for concurrent rehabilitation programmes to stimulate auto-control systems.

SPASTICITY IN SKELETAL MUSCULATURE

Persistent hypertonia and hyper-reflexia following a stroke affects ongoing performance. If the inhibitory procedures in positioning and handling fail to contain it while auto-inhibition is re-programmed, then other means need to be explored.

One of the two anti-spasticity agents usually prescribed is **baclofen** (marketed as **Lioresal**), which is believed to possess a GABA-mimetic (gamma-amino-butyric acid, an inhibitory neurotransmitter) activity which enhances presynaptic inhibition of spinal motoneurons. Because it acts at spinal level to decrease enhanced monosynaptic reflex activity, there is a centrally-acting element which, in older people particularly, can induce an initial 'muzziness'. This wears off after a few days on a minimal dose (5 mg a day, for instance), and when it does the dose can be slowly increased. It can also enhance possible post-stroke epilepsy, and should be used with caution if there is already a history of epilepsy.

It may interact (by further lowering blood pressure) with antihypertensives (prescribed for high blood pressure), tricyclic antidepressants, some of the non-steroidal anti-inflammatory preparations such as ibuprofen (prescribed for arthritis, painful joints, etc.) and levodopa (for Parkinson's disease). If still appropriate, dosage usually commences at 15 mg daily, divided into three doses (5 mg, three times a day). The tablets are 10 mg each and tiny, so halving them is quite tricky! It is available in liquid form for 5 ml doses, which solves this problem (also easier for people who have difficulty swallowing tablets). The daily dose can be increased every 3 days until reduction in muscle tone is just sufficient to allow function – usually to a maximum of about 60 mg daily.

Withdraw the drug gradually (don't just stop the tablets), otherwise spasticity is rapidly aggravated and this will obscure the true state.

The other common anti-spasticity agent, **dantrolene sodium** (marketed as **Dantrium**), acts directly on skeletal muscle tissue beyond the neuromuscular junction by inhibiting the release and uptake of intracellular calcium (which is necessary for muscle contraction). Because of this it should be used with caution in patients with impaired pulmonary function and patients with severely impaired cardiac function due to myocardial disease. It has a potentially hepatoxic action (long periods on the higher dosage), so liver function tests should be performed before starting to establish a baseline, again six weeks later, and thereafter at the physician's discretion. The starting dose is 25 mg daily (the capsules contain either 25 mg or 100 mg dantrolene sodium) increased slowly, week by week, to a maximum of 400 mg daily after seven weeks, and titrated according to need. As with baclofen, some early dizziness and occasionally nausea and/or diarrhoea may be experienced. If the nausea or diarrhoea persists, then reduce the dose or withdraw the drug. The top dose should not be maintained in the long term – lengthy use can result in generalized muscle weakness, which will further increase the problems for stroke-survivors!

If spasticity is still markedly affecting function, then return to the starting dose and begin to introduce baclofen.

As baclofen and dantrolene sodium act independently and at different levels, they can be used together in cases of severe spasticity.

The use of these drugs does sound pretty last-ditch, but in fact either or both can be very effective. In the short-term, spasticity can be reduced while auto-inhibitory systems are being established. If this remains impaired, then functional performance in many cases can be maintained with longer term use subject to regular review.

Benzodiazepines (such as Diazepam) increase GABA activity at cerebral level, and therefore reduce the activity of anterior horn cells at the spinal level, and are effective skeletal muscle relaxants for generalized 'spasm' in many neurological conditions – but **not** for the unilateral hypertonic musculature of stroke.

They relax all the skeletal musculature rendering the recipient generally hypotonic but without reducing tone significantly in the S musculature, with the result that more effort is required to function which stimulates further unilateral hyper-reflexia with hypertonia. They also produce a feeling of tiredness and slight 'remoteness' which affects concentration and makes it more difficult to initiate movement. Continence can also be affected, which is distressing.

They are also used for sedation and to promote a 'good night's sleep'. For Strokes who suffer with nighttime flexor spasms these preparations offer some respite, but any sedatives tend to carry-over and impair daytime functional performance, so they should be carefully monitored and the dosage prioritized accordingly.

DROOLING

Excessive saliva (not poor containment of saliva), if really profuse, can sometimes be reduced with atropine or other drugs with antimuscarinic properties. Beware of precipitating urinary retention and constipation, i.e. do not use long-term.

INCONTINENCE

The antimuscarinic drugs such as Micturin block parasympathetic control, and may be used to treat urinary frequency, urgency and incontinence.

Cholinergics (such as Bethanechol) and anticholinesterases (such as Distigmine) are used to treat urinary retention. They promote bladder voiding by increasing the tone of the detrusor muscle.

11.5 MODERN TECHNOLOGY

This is a remarkably interesting time in which to be working! The 'advancing edge of medicine' is really pushing out the barriers of science and, conversely, scientific exploration in other directions is contributing enormously to developments in the medical world. One stroke-survivor with whom I worked had, for instance, been a design consultant working with international aerospace programmes; he linked the background research and development of heat-seeking missiles to the emerging concept of extended closed-loop 'pursuit' control of movement.

The picturing or scanning of live brain tissue through techniques like MRI and CT enhances the diagrams and models derived from post-mortem studies, and more recently computerized anatomical atlases have illuminated medical education.

An interactive dissection-like volume model derived from 3D-imaging modalities (such as CT, MRI, US and confocal microscopy) has been developed at the Institute of Mathematics and Computer Science in Medicine and the Department of Neuroanatomy, Hamburg (Hohne et al., 1992). This not only gives the teaching (and learning) of anatomy a 3D-visible knowledge base, but can be used clinically to allow a pre-surgical pictorial exploration into the structural relationships and potential hazards which will be presented at the time of actual surgery for each case, for instance, both for specific reference and also in preparation for possible alternative procedures for locating and doing what needs to be done in all eventualities.

The screen images of the brain at work obtained through **PET** (Positron Emission Tomography) are real rather than representational. PET uses a harmless mixture of glucose with a tiny amount of radioactive tracer compound injected into the bloodstream. The most active neurons require the most glucose, and therefore the PET scan acts rather like a Geiger counter in measuring the amount of radioactivity as the labelled glucose is taken up by the brain cells. The results are colour-graphically computed to show the different levels of neural activity in the brain. By comparing PET scans of 'normal' individuals with those of neurologically impaired individuals a variety of problems can be identified.

Of many advances in micro-processor technology applicable to rehabilitation, few appear to be relevant to stroke other than as adjuncts to different but concurrent needs. Two modalities that can be gainfully employed are 'prompting' devices and electrical neuromuscular stimulation.

The electrically-induced movement systems FES (functional electrical stimulation) are more appropriate to lower motor neuron injuries than to lesions in the brain itself.

BIOFEEDBACK

This form of personal feedback draws particular attention to specific problem factors, and enhances awareness and concentration to overcome them. The devices are quite costly, so investigate manufacturers' claims and assess potential need before purchasing. Not all Strokes will respond with sufficient improvement in performance to warrant generalized use.

A **pressure pad** in the shoe will beep on heel-strike – or beep until the heel pressure cuts it off. There are several designs and options. The pads do take space (so shoes need to be roomy) and tend to be temperamental in use.

Weight-sensor footplates and a visual monitor screen with colour-coded signals (and an optional auditory signal) have proved effective in the treatment of abnormal stance symmetry and weight-transference (Sackley et al., 1992). The design allows for free intervention by therapists working to facilitate normal posture and transference of weight in standing and stepping. The response through both footplates indicates anomalies in weight-bearing (between the S foot and the N foot, and between heels and toes) and prompts active correction. The same model has an optional 'seat' which indicates weight distribution in sitting. If funds are limited, try two bathroom scales, one for each foot!

There are several devices marketed for the sports and leisure industry which could be utilized in stroke rehabilitation, in particular those which offer a **moving platform** to stimulate dynamic postural adjustment and equilibrium reactions. One version designed for the rehabilitation of skiing injuries comprises a tension-loaded skate gliding on an arc-shaped platform, and can be used in standing and sitting, and also for upper limb stabilizing techniques. Obviously any non-medical apparatus requires extra care if used with stroke-disabled clients. Safety must be ensured and precautionary grab-rails, harness and so on provided in addition to personal supervision.

Specifically-designed **computer games** and programmes help concentration, scanning and dexterity, and can also assist the organization of executive planning skills for certain cognitive impairments. It provides a more adult exercise than jigsaw puzzles, and for many older clients it is an interesting learning experience which could be developed further. One inattentive very elderly Stroke with unilateral neglect was introduced to a computer to compose and write shopping lists; she now owns her own Computer and is the pride of the neighbourhood.

Computer-studies departments in Sixth-form colleges and the like are often delighted to design appropriate software as a special project.

ELECTRICAL NEUROMUSCULAR STIMULATION

As with all intervention to do with the rehabilitation of stroke, studies and trials to date regarding outcomes are inconclusive. However, customized programmes for selected clients – those with hypertonic and hyper-reflexic musculature, for instance – do seem to be effective. Spasticity can be reduced, giving hands-on intervention a chance to rebuild functional activity and to sustain more normal movement. The beneficial effects are seen and felt generally, not just in the treated limb, and there are few adverse reactions (unlike drug therapy). Excluded from some of these programmes are people with demand-type cardiac pacemakers or those with cardiac arrhythmias; read the literature and question the manufacturers if in doubt. Physiotherapy core expertise includes electrotherapy, so this is one of their range of treatments.

Discussed here is a technology developed from the work on neuro-muscular plasticity. These units differ from other electrical stimulation models in their basic specifications.

Suggested for use in stroke rehabilitation programmes are **dual-channel stimulators** offering the choice of synchronous or alternate operation in a very low frequency range: 1–99 pulses per second (pps, Hz). The asymmetrical biphasic pulse width can be adjusted between 20–400 microseconds (μs), the actual range depending on the inbuilt parameters, and the pulse itself can be set to sub-pulse or extended-pulse mode in certain models.

An adjustable stimulation/relaxation cycle is necessary to prevent overstimulation of muscle tissue. The relaxation period should be as long as the stimulation period to allow reactive hyperaemia to disperse. Once the frequency is raised to a level which produces a tetanic contraction, it may be more appropriate to enlist a longer stimulation to allow a movement to occur – the client is required to produce a voluntary contraction during this stimulatory period, and to consciously relax the muscle group between stimulations. Amplitude is controllable by the operator or user each time.

Some units come pre-programmed for specific output, some are programmable by the operator for wide-ranging specific and selective use. Most offer a small battery-operated unit suitable for domestic application under the physiotherapist's guidance, and some companies offer leasing facilities.

The selection of parameters needs to be scrupulously assessed for each individual and relates directly to the particular effect required.

Frequency

Below 5 pps to introduce the stimulus to a nerve-muscle situation which may not respond immediately or may not have functioned for a period of years. For example, 3 pps is the natural firing frequency of the fusimotor pathways which control the muscle spindles and initiate the movement sequence. It is used as an introductory frequency for spasticity. It is also within the frequency window for pain relief programmes (TENS/TNS, transcutaneous electrical nerve stimulation) and for general relaxation.

5–15 pps is selected to improve muscle tone. These frequencies may be used for long periods (up to three hours a day, and up to ten hours a day for specific protocols). For example, the natural firing frequency of the slow oxidative (SO) muscle fibres is 10 pps; electrical stimulation will improve the muscle's resistance to fatigue by improving its capillary bed density and increasing its ability to handle oxygen break-down.

15–25 pps promotes endurance in muscle tissue. This is the natural frequency band for the fast oxidative/glycolytic fibres. Treatment can be given for one hour a day.

30–40 pps will recruit the fast glycolytic fibres and is selected for strengthening muscles. These frequencies are used to gain tetanic contractions and therefore require the recipient to contract and relax in time with the stimulation/relaxation cycle. Treatment here should be given for short periods only – ten minutes or so – to prevent undue fatigue.

Channel selection

Alternate channel mode reproduces agonist/antagonist muscle activity. It is used in the protocols for spasticity, to stimulate reciprocal innervation and inhibition.

Simultaneous channel mode allows for the reproduction of whole limb movement in one direction (extension of elbow and wrist, for instance) and synergic muscle activity.

Pulse width

Pulse width selection is made according to the depth of penetration required – the shorter the width the more comfortable and superficial the treatment received. For example, for superficial muscles of the face or hand – 80 μs; for arm muscles, 100–150 μs; for leg muscles, about 200 μs.

All treatments should be adjusted to fall within the recipient's natural tolerance levels (maybe 200 μs for the arm, and so on).

Variations within the available pulse width band cannot adversely affect the treatment.

(These parameters are based on the literature provided by DMI Medical Ltd (1989) and are quoted with their permission.)

All treatments and changes in programming must be subject to the supervision and approval of a qualified physiotherapist who is experienced in the use of these units. The selected programmes should be recorded in detail, with changes in client performance, for evaluation. This can also enable new protocols to be developed.

Electrical neuromuscular stimulation in the treatment of CVA seems, as yet, only to be significant when the reactivated systems are reinforced by the physiological stressing of human endeavour, and so is really a strategy to facilitate normal movement, which then needs to be utilized to sustain ongoing normal movement. The application of this and other modalities to neurological rehabilitation, as in the studies of EMNS in lower limb spasticity (Shindo and Jones, 1987) and Bell's palsy (Farragher, 1987) – to create change by trophic engineering in the form of electrical neuromuscular stimulation – is an epic breakthrough with enormous potential that has yet to be fully explored.

Look to the future with vigour and not with fondness on the past.

(*Geoffrey Kidd*)

REFERENCES

DMI Medical Instruments (1989), *Instruction Manual*, DMI Medical Instruments, Wigan, UK.

Farragher, D.J. (1987) Eutrophic stimulation for Bell's Palsy. *Clinical Rehabilitation*, **1**, 265–71.

Gildenberg, P.L. (1984) Myelotomy and percutaneous cordotomy for the treatment of cancer pain. *Applied Neurophysiology*, **47**, 208–15.

Hohne, K.H., Bomans, M., Riemer, M., Schubert, R., Tiede, U. and Lierse, W. (1992) A volume-based anatomical atlas. *IEEE Computer Graphics and Applications*, July, 72–8.

Parragon Books (1993) *Medicines*, Parragon, Bristol.

Rawlings, C., Rossitch, E. and Nashold, B.S. (1992) The history of neurosurgical procedures for the relief of pain. *Surgical Neurology*, **38**, 454–63.

Sackley, C.M., Baguley, B.I., Gent, S. and Hodgson, P. (1992) The use of a balance performance monitor in the treatment of weight-bearing and weight-transference problems after stroke. *Physiotherapy*, **78**(12), 907–12.

Sampson, J.H. and Nashold, B.S. (1992) Facial pain due to vascular lesions of the brain stem relieved by dorsal root entry zone lesions in the nucleus caudalis. *Journal of Neurosurgery*, **77**, 473–5.

Simpson, B.A. (1991) Spinal cord stimulation in 60 cases of intractable pain. *Journal of Neurology, Neurosurgery and Psychiatry*, **54**, 196–9.

Shindo, N. and Jones, R. (1987) Reciprocal patterned electrical stimulation of the lower limbs in severe spasticity. *Physiotherapy*, **73**(10), 579–82.

Young, R.F. (1990) Clinical experience with radiofrequency and laser DREZ lesions. *Journal of Neurosurgery*, **72**, 715–20.

The responsibility 12

The most melancholy of human reflections, perhaps, is that, on the whole, it is a question whether the benevolence of mankind does most good or harm.
(Walter Bagehot)

Neuromuscular plasticity determines that people with a suddenly-acquired neurological disorder such as a stroke are totally susceptible to change from that moment on.

I am currently formulating a theory with a speech and language therapy colleague, Dr Wayne Wilson, which suggests that the central nervous system response to acute trauma once the biological shock has subsided – or even as part of the 'shock' response – is the initiation of an immediate 'emergency repair' process which cobbles together the available parts of any systems which can be utilized for the continuation of an approximately functional state. We hypothesize that this patching is of such a high order that future 'darning', as in carefully-orchestrated rehabilitation, can only take second place – necessitating laborious volitional effort in order to perform accurately each and every time. This would account for the apparent immutability of some abnormal patterns of movement and speech following stroke.

Recovery patterns in speech and language seem to be successfully sustained and improved upon following discharge from therapy. Maybe this is because speech and language are seen as the vital element in all human contact to ensure self-preservation and social contact, and re-acquisition is therefore strongly self-motivated.

The recovery of motor behaviour is more of a minefield. For many Strokes, high standards in performance reached during active physical therapy programmes are not often maintained after the period of treatment has ended. Sometimes this is attributable to over-indulgent personal carers, but in most cases it could be because the natural tendency is to run on 'automatic' in the domestic environment – which could be to return to the immediately post-stroke reorganized networking.

Even disregarding this theoretical explanation the facts as presented to date are indisputable:

- the rehabilitation of stroke must start from the very moment of trauma to salvage and protect the normality of future behaviour patterns, and to prevent the establishing of abnormality and 'learned non-use';
- for Strokes who have missed this early intervention, and for those with more severe focal disruption, exact and intense physiological stressing must be applied in order to recover and maintain any normality.

Every person bears equal and ongoing responsibility for enabling as well as for disabling every Stroke individual in their care. This simple statement raises two issues which need a little more analysis.

Adulthood brings responsibilities, for 'self' and for others (whether humans, pets or pot plants), which give purpose to existence. To deprive another adult – the Stroke – of responsibility contributes to their deprivation of a sense of adulthood. Chapter 9 has already discussed the need to include the Stroke as a 'partner in care': no-one can be motivated whose present and future are exclusively in the control of others. Older people are particularly at risk – as work and family responsibilities decrease there are fewer needs to 'keep going'. If personal and domestic responsibility is then taken over by other people, however well intentioned, there is nothing purposeful left for them to do. So the responsibility of all carers, both professional and domestic, is also to allow the Stroke to be responsible, to feel in control – as discreetly as possible, and surreptitiously if necessary – in as many ways as can be devised, to recreate a sense of purpose in a life made seemingly useless 'at a stroke'.

Caring can be interpreted several ways. It can mean:

- caretaking – looking after in a non-reciprocal situation, such as exists in many long-stay residential and nursing homes;
- caregiving – implies non-reciprocal assistance where appropriate;
- concern for another's wellbeing.

Caring in terms of stroke should mean concern, and involve a reciprocal relationship. The following comments have been collected from various sources during meetings and conferences. Some are attributable and some are not, but all are gratefully acknowledged here:

Many families try to insulate stroke patients from everyday stress and do far too much for them. This hinders their chances of making a full recovery and encourages them in living a 'sick' role.

The hermetic nature of family life fashions the way we become dependent on other peoples dependency.

...the de-skilling of family care.

(Eric Wilkes, Emeritus Professor of Community Care and General Practice, Sheffield University)

This last quote refers to the protective professionalism which excludes family involvement.

The next piece was written about dementia, but seems equally relevant to stroke and attitudes to the severely disabled generally:

...concept of dementia is itself part of a broader belief system; one that is widespread throughout the developed world – that reflects the central significance given to autonomy and independence as the ultimate criteria for adulthood. We find dementia to be a tragedy because it represents a tragic way of growing old and dying. The tragedy lies in the loss of control, of agency, and thereby of adult status ... Old age out of control, how frightening. But dementia is a tragedy in part because we give such central importance to the individual and to individual relationships ... Dirty houses can be cleaned, wandering people can be returned home, hands can be held and foolishness laughed at ... What a way to go, we may think. But it seems to me that there are many worse ways of leaving this singular life of ours: dying bravely rather than dying foolishly may turn out to be an over-estimated virtue.

(Gilleard, 1991)

The **medical model** is about 'patients' and 'management' of the disease process – a three-tier system of 'them' and 'us' and 'it'. The stroke-survivor in a rehabilitation programme is really little different from someone attending a sports centre to get fit. Stroke is not an illness, and stroke management is more about the management of the team than the person. It should be the Stroke who manages the stroke, utilizing the facilities offered by the team. The next sequence is of comments made by stroke-survivors of the medical model, to further highlight these issues:

Simple things become impossible ... getting hopelessly entangled in my shirt ... People talking about me as they would a child – my power gone, vanished ...

(Vincent Hepp, three years after his stroke)

*It is companionable to share some of the day-to-day triumphs and despairs ... terribly cheerful people are no help at all ... How fragile we all are, and I felt so safe and well. Now I've been knocked down – and that is what is difficult – to be so **suddenly** old – a radical change of life.*

(May Sarton, 1988)

Where is this? It's like a geriatric ward in here.
(An older stroke patient on entering hospital: she had indeed been admitted directly to a long-stay general elderly care ward)

...it helped a great deal when they [her husband and daughter] were able to tell me they knew what I meant because you had explained what was going on in my mind and the difficulty I was having in retrieving the words – it meant I didn't have to worry about being unable to explain my problem and it allowed me to relax and therefore progress ...

This last extract is from a letter written nine months after an apparently very severe stroke. The relatives had been told, just days after the stroke, that she would never walk or talk again, was intellectually impaired, and in view of her continuing incontinence (catheterized within 24 hours of admission to the hospital) she would have to go into long-term nursing home care as further recovery could not be expected. Their friends telephoned the author for advice. The family succeeded in getting her transferred to their nearest stroke unit and, four months later, she was discharged home, walking, talking, continent and with full movement in her R arm. The family had participated in her rehabilitation throughout. Her daughter has written:

I consider the professionals are all too anxious to be negative – they say you must be realistic ... When relatives are putting in so much personal effort they need encouragement – the worst thing is to take away their hope.

Perhaps professional pessimism merely reflects the (quite justifiable) professional sense of inadequacy, compounded in this case by a local ignorance of stroke and of specialist stroke rehabilitation, but early judgements are never accurate (though sometimes self-fulfilling if rehabilitation is withdrawn as a result!) and are therefore inexcusable. The same Stroke is now back to completing the *Daily Telegraph* cross-word, and has further confounded the family by displaying an entirely new ability to process quite complex mathematical calculations 'in her head', discovered while watching a TV quiz show (pre-stroke, even checking till-receipts was chancy, they say).

Obviously not all stroke-survivors recover to such a dramatic degree, nevertheless the potential for improvement is always present and this must always be fully recognized. This chapter discusses:

12.1 Ethics
12.2 Roles
12.3 Community groups and organizations
12.4 Practical advice

12.1 ETHICS

Every profession has its own written code of ethics. Confidentiality may seem jeopardized in team situations, but each member of the professional team is bound by a similar code so the exchange of necessary information should remain unrestricted. It is vitally important for realistic planning to know if a partner is unsupportive, but details regarding marital history are not, even if recounted to several persons by one or both of the individuals concerned.

The unwritten codes of conduct and social behaviour, also, should be adhered to throughout!

INTERVENTION

Human rights are not always recognizable in day-to-day situations: the dividing line between 'intervention' and 'intrusion' is all too easily crossed. Rehabilitation of stroke is a very hands-on process involving much physical 'moulding' of the trunk and limbs and facilitative handling, and assessment by feeling for specific muscle responses to changes in posture. Constant observation (for the same purposes) can seem intrusive too.

Be impersonal but natural, introduce everything gradually until the Stroke is reassured that such invasion of personal privacy is purely rehabilitative. Explain, discuss, include, involve and communicate.

Dependency is an inviduous growth which feeds on caretaking sustained caregiving. Ensure that there is plenty of time each day for the Stroke to enjoy actual personal privacy – to replenish the sense of self and to learn to cope with freedom.

Attitudes do have to be positive – but not bullish! The utmost consideration must be given to:

- dignity, e.g. clothing, personal hygiene, presentation, personal space;
- respect, for adulthood and for individuality;
- partnership in care;
- enablement and empowerment;
- reciprocal relationships;
- quality of life,

and these considerations apply equally to the carers themselves (professional and personal) and to the Strokes.

The **invasion of personal privacy** includes unwarranted intrusion – from excessive observation to unnecessary hands-on – from over-familiarity of address (e.g. first names for some, generic labels like 'granny' for others) to participating uninvited in private occasions when family or friends are present for instance (or removing the Stroke for treatment during a long-awaited visit). Always try to arrange times for treatment, and for family involvement or discussion, to mutual satisfaction in advance.

Invasion of personal privacy also includes being subjected to continuous music (usually chosen, without consultation, by staff), whether it be the latest chart-toppers or golden oldies on a perpetually repeating cycle.

Video filming and photography for rehabilitation purposes requires the voluntary agreement of the individual concerned. If the results – in whole or in part – are to be shown outside the immediate rehabilitation environment (for teaching purposes, workshop or for publication in any format), then the reasons must be clearly given and comprehended and written permission must be obtained first (or a statement, knowingly signed).

'Personality clashes' and stress require appropriate intervention as soon as the problem is identified, and this is important for staff and clients and families alike (therapists and nurses could be easier to replace than partners!).

PROFESSIONAL INTERVENTION

Stroke survivors are highly individual human beings linked only by a diagnosis. A stroke produces impairment of generally accepted 'norms'. Each stroke produces an unforecastable range and degree of disability. Professional intervention therefore has to be somewhat *ad hoc* with all the inherent and attendant risks.

Iatrogenesis is defined in Taber's *Cyclopedic Medical Dictionary* as any adverse mental or physical condition induced in a patient by the effects of treatment by a physician or surgeon. The term further implies that such effects could have been avoided by proper and judicious care on the part of the practitioner (El-Din, 1991). An American study in the general medical service of a university hospital found that 36% of 815 patients had an iatrogenic illness – and length of stay was a correlated factor. Dr El-Din draws attention to the implications of iatrogenesis in other areas of work and advocates precise analysis and careful prescription, client-centred goals, and documentation related to outcomes for accurate evaluation.

In rehabilitation, iatrogenesis could result from actual treatment (including the use of poorly-understood, unnecessary or inappropriate techniques) as well as a lack of – or ineffectual – treatment.

Sins of omission relevant to clinical practice are:

- delay in initiating rehabilitation;
- avoidable delay – or reluctance – in referring a client to a more appropriate source of expertise;
- insufficient or omitted communication with other involved persons;
- ignoring, not analysing, or delaying the investigation of abnormal or impoverished-normal signs, symptoms and reactions;
- apathy regarding the acquisition and heuristic application of any new knowledge or understanding which could improve the rehabilitation of stroke-survivors.

Traditional timetables do need revising and updating in their philosophy of care. Hospital ward, therapy department and professional input routines must be flexible enough to be client-led, and communication is vital. For example, washing and dressing doesn't have to be rushed through by the night-shift nurses before breakfast. Physiotherapists, as well as nurses and occupational therapists, should be able to absorb this into a rehabilitation session on the ward (Chapter 13 details the procedures). Therapy is not confined to a therapy department.

Physiotherapists who find themselves stuck with unprogressing physical ability in a Stroke who appears to have a good potential for further recovery, need advice from the occupational therapists who specialize in perceptual problems. The author was once refused this, on the grounds that 'the results of perceptual tests are confidential and exclusive to the occupational therapist and the doctor', which complicated and delayed that client's rehabilitation (however, this incident did precipitate the author's enrolment on the first available course in cognitive neuropsychology!) Another therapist, concerned about a client's underlying cardiac condition, was refused access to medical notes by a ward sister for much the same reasons.

Nurses face similar obstacles: screened-off by curtains while a therapist works with a Stroke at the bedside, and seldom given time to visit the therapy departments, they are then pilloried for failing to reinforce the rehabilitation programme.

Traditionally, only occupational therapists work closely with the social workers for a planned discharge from hospital, but all team members need to contribute their appropriate areas of expertise. Physiotherapists could and should be more involved, predictive assessment being part of their core expertise and an essential cost-effective step, too, when structural alterations or expensive equipment are under discussion. A stairlift or a downstairs bathroom may not be required if further rehabilitation can be arranged (domiciliary from choice or as an out-patient, with interim measures in place such as a commode and downstairs daybed).

It's not surprising that stroke rehabilitation has been so confused and generally ineffectual for so long – it is built on shifting sand. A standard policy has to be tight enough to uphold acceptable standards (and these are themselves subject to change!), yet loose enough to allow for the necessary pragmatism in such an individualized condition. Inter-disciplinary teamwork is poorly understood. Professional intervention in many instances has remained unstructured and incomplete, isolated behind professional boundaries, and even basic techniques are still mistakenly withheld from adoption into common core skills in many areas.

12.2 ROLES

Who is Sylvia? What is she?

(A popular Edwardian ballad)

Responsibility in stroke rehabilitation encompasses not only rehabilitation of the stroke-survivor, but also the acquisition and sharing of relevant knowledge. Teamwork has already been explored; this section identifies some members of the team.

The **nursing** role in Stroke management includes the primary enabling of normal functional activity, using common-core skills.

The titles of **therapists** are self-explanatory and should be understood already: they share this primary responsibility as well.

Other personnel (porters, ambulance personnel, domestic staff, technicians, support workers, community workers, etc.), family and friends also share this responsibility.

The role of the **doctor** is seen as diagnostic, investigative and prescriptive in terms of medication and intervention. Tradition gives an advisory and coordinating role too, but this is often unsatisfactory because of the degree of commitment required – few doctors can give sufficient time to collect and disseminate such a wealth of information. Nevertheless, 'patients' and relatives expect the doctors to be gurus and their every word is carved on tablets of stone. To promote optimism without compromising realistic expectations depends upon effective interdisciplinary communication; doctors in company with all the members of a multidisciplinary team must be prepared to admit their limitations and accept the necessity to refer on for appropriate advice or intervention.

Social workers have a more ambiguous profile, traditionally bridging the gap between hospital and community care and acting as the advocate for the client as well as advising on welfare issues – and processing benefits both monetary and material – such as rehousing, structural alterations or equipment – to enable clients to remain in, or return to, their own homes, or to be appropriately resettled in a place of their own choosing.

The role of a medical social worker – taken from conversations with experienced colleagues who have a special interest in working with stroke-disabled clients and their families – is described here in some detail because their philosophy, of enablement leading to empowerment, embodies the entire rehabilitation process and raises awareness of the many other factors which concern the stroke-survivor and their relatives.

The medical social worker is the team member whose particular role is to help clients to work out their personal and social problems resulting from the stroke. People come from every section of the community, and all need help:

- both emotionally and practically in accepting their disability, to come to terms with their own frailty and to review their lifestyle prior to discharge;
- to cope with fear of disability and of dying;
- to adjust to an institutional organization and to understand and relate to professional intervention.

Clients include:

- people who always have problems (of inadequacy, deprivation, delinquency) which become more pressing when illness is added to them;
- people who have previously managed to keep going under their own resources, but for whom illness is the 'last straw' so they can no longer cope;
- people, previously highly competent, for whom the illness itself constitutes the actual problem and who find it difficult to relate to needing help.

The initial interview is the most important – to gain the client's permission for the involvement of others, to introduce freedom of choice, frankness and flexibility, respect and trust – so that when action is required in the handling of personal matters it is understood that this will be done with confidentiality and efficiency.

It is necessary to:

- build a relationship with the client on a one-to-one basis;
- be a good listener, to clients and their relatives, in order to build up a complete picture of their relationships and attitudes;
- gain insight into previous lifestyle and interests in order to ensure that all possible stimulation can be given appropriately, to pave the way for a return to active life;
- allow expression of anger, frustration, and fears about the future;
- make realistic plans, stage by stage.

Patience, courtesy, kindness and the privacy of a quiet interview room are basic factors in guiding and counselling, and also for enlisting assistance from previously untapped (or hitherto unapproachable) sources. The social worker plays a vital role in liaising between dispersed team members including Local Authority departments, relatives, neighbours and voluntary helpers. Practical measures are taken to ensure that bills are paid, pensions drawn, statutory benefits understood and applied for, and that the house is clean and warm with food and assistance available on discharge home. It is sometimes necessary to dispel unrealistic expectations in both relatives and client about their capabilities. Older Strokes and their relatives may need advice regarding the possibility of continuing care and its provision.

No firm decisions should be taken until the team has collectively agreed a final analysis of the predicted outcome of rehabilitation. Many Strokes can and do manage to live in their own homes with community support; if their home has already been sold this negates all sense of purpose and adds to the feelings of bereavement. This is particularly tragic if it is later found to have been an unnecessary step.

It is important to assess the home situation as soon as possible. The first home visit – with the client, a therapist (either OT or physio., both if possible) and a relative if appropriate – will, at an early stage, set a baseline for realistic planning. The social worker has all the information needed regarding alternative housing and the provision of structural alterations, adaptations and continuing care packages, together with the availability of financial aid from statutory and charitable sources for these purposes.

Clients are encouraged and assisted to share in (and take responsibility for, wherever possible) all planning for their future. Support given is always non-judgemental, and their need to make their own decisions is always recognized.

Legal advisors may need to be contacted and invited to meet with relevant members of the team to gain an accurate picture of the client's competence in order to protect the client's interests, if someone is requesting power of attorney to take over financial control of the client's affairs, for instance. Language-impaired clients are particularly at risk in these situations.

The younger Strokes may need urgent intervention, to organize continuity of income for mortgage repayments and/or other financial commitments, and to ensure the continuation of as normal a life as possible for their children. Children of all ages should be kept in touch – literally – with a parent in hospital; they are surprisingly matter-of-fact. Even small children can see, and start to understand and play a practical part in, the progress towards recovery.

Other home visits are arranged as relevant, as circumstances change and rehabilitation progresses, to ensure that the final discharge plans are up-to-date and appropriate. Social workers may coordinate the planned discharge and also arrange and monitor ongoing support and aftercare. A visit to the client's home a few days after discharge is important: this is the time when the reality of personal disability (which may have become acceptable in the hospital environment) is acutely realized and reassurance urgently needed.

The transition from a hospital or housebound situation to resuming a normal lifestyle in the community can be difficult. Voluntary organizations, clubs, day centres and workshops can be contacted, and visits and outings arranged as the formal rehabilitation programmes are scaled down.

Respite care – short admissions at regular intervals into residential or nursing home accommodation – can provide relief for family carers.

Follow-up visits ensure that independence aids and gadgets are still appropriate – regular review is needed to allow for changes in functional ability.

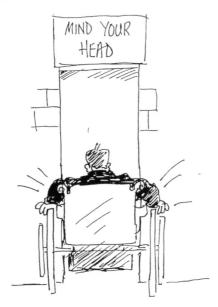

Survey accessibility before outings ... (Reproduced with permission from the artist Geoffrey Whitehead.)

12.3 COMMUNITY GROUPS AND ORGANIZATIONS

Many Strokes and families are unaware of the existence of the many support and self-help groups in the neighbourhood. Information about these should be freely available from several sources: Social Services, libraries, Community Health Councils, appropriate national organizations and specific advisory groups such as the Council for Voluntary Services and the Stroke Association in UK and the local Physically Handicapped Associations. It is recommended that a local survey (formal or informal) is undertaken so that details can be offered to people who are unable to access the sources for themselves. Some schools are delighted to do this as part of a social studies programme, and can often produce a leaflet or booklet listing the results. 'Environmental Accessibility for Disabled (or Less-Able) Persons' is another useful project!

Most national organizations have local branches – if there is not one in the immediate area, then advice or assistance is sometimes given to start one.

Groups specifically for stroke-survivors are often more supportive than those with a mixed membership of physically disabled: the problems of stroke are complex and Strokes frequently feel socially embarrassed for quite a long time. Some enthusiastic Strokes, families or friends could be assisted to form a local self-help community stroke group if there is not one already – or to open another if needs are not being met; some clubs are distinctly 'care-giving' and merely reinforce the sense of dependency (very unstimulating). The sharing of experience and strategies for coping with persons in similar predicaments is valuable and therapeutic for the Stroke, and for relatives and friends, and necessary fundraising creates a mutual sense of purpose in everybody concerned.

Ideally, community-based or domiciliary professionals could visit such groups to work with clients and families in this unstructured social setting, to advise on DIY rehabilitation strategies and to promote further independence. One-to-one relationships can be broadened and audience participation is sympathetic, supportive and fruitful. For many clients the rehabilitation programmes given to them in their own home or in hospital departments remain associated with just those situations, and carry-over into other settings is seldom implemented. Dynamic postural control can be more usefully maintained and improved if the need is recognized and worked on during an art class or while laying a table for lunch.

Organizations such as Cruse in UK offer specialized bereavement counselling. Most counsellors have themselves suffered bereavement, many through long-term or terminal illness of partners – ask for someone who is experienced in working with the grief of physical disability and its implications.

Housing organizations and cooperatives often include purpose-built accommodation for the physically handicapped in their properties, some offering community rooms and meals, or wardens on-site. Supervised flatlets are sometimes available – for independence trials, or for couples to gain confidence in coping – if these facilities cannot be provided in a rehabilitation centre.

Rehabilitation centres are in short supply in many areas, but longer-term residential rehabilitation is essential in certain cases where ongoing recovery is predictable or management of severe residual disablement can be improved upon. Always try for a place in these circumstances.

12.4 PRACTICAL ADVICE

This section is a random collection of helpful hints and suggestions, gathered over the years from Strokes themselves, their families and friends, professionals and non-professionals. Their value has been well-proven and they deserve general recognition!

- Many Strokes are reluctant to face themselves in a mirror – imagined or perceived disablement creates anxiety and heightens the sense of personal disfigurement. Prevention is always simpler than the cure: it is important to introduce the natural use of a familiar small hand-held or free-standing tabletop mirror into everyday functional activity from the first day – for shaving, hair-tidying, applying make-up if it is used, and so on. Encourage its use for remedial purposes too – simple exercises to restore tonus to facial musculature, for instance.

- A duvet is easier to cope with than a clutter of tucked-in bedclothes, which can make getting in and out of bed quite arduous and also obstruct free movement in bed.
- Toilet paper is best provided in flat pack single-sheet dispensers; pulling sections from a roll is almost impossible with one hand, unless several sheets are first unrolled and rewound once or twice around the holder itself in order to fix it firmly. The toilet-roll holders or dispensers should be sited to the N side (on both sides in hospitals or Homes). Disposable moistened tissues such as 'Baby-Wipes' are excellent for final cleansing after going to the loo – both for private parts and for hands afterwards – and most brands can be flushed down the toilet. They are designed for sensitive places, are unperfumed and usually biodegradable, and ensure a hygienic atmosphere in personal and extra-personal space until the next proper wash.
- Portable and discreet forms of urinal or slipper-type bedpans allay anxiety on long journeys.
- Leisure-wear, such as jogging or tracksuits, are comfortable and attractive for most people to wear. They are easy to get on and off, and the elasticated waists simplify toileting too. Men may need the front seam of the trousers unstitched below the elastic – trying to hold the waistband down while coping with everything else is impossible with one hand (there is usually plenty of fabric gathered at the waist which effectively screens across). Ordinary trousers may need the front opening extended down to the inner leg seam.
- Footwear should be comfortable and supportive: allow for any oedema and bandaging or strapping. 'Trainers' in a larger size are a useful interim measure. Elastic laces don't give enough support. There are several canny methods for doing up ordinary laces using only one hand, ask an occupational therapist. Velcro fastenings are an option, and shoe-repairers will sometimes add these to replace laces.
- Mittens are easier to put on than gloves.
- Simple accessories like an across-the-shoulder or waistband bag for carrying personal items, an easily-accessible purse, a discreet cover for a 'bottle' or urine bag, and a necessary arm-support (Figure 10.26) made in a coordinating fabric to blend in with clothing, all contribute to confident living.
- Shopping trips need to be included in rehabilitation programmes for most individuals. The ability to cope – with purses and handbags and money, to choose items, to stop *en route* for a seat, a cup of coffee,

and maybe a visit to an unfamiliar lavatory – eases a return to life in the outside world. (A preliminary survey for accessibility should be undertaken before setting out!)

- People need something to do – so much time is spent just sitting and waiting. Any stimulation, mental or physical, is vitally important to revive interest in life after a stroke. Organized group activities play a part, but a personal creative or constructive (or just plain enjoyable) occupation is even more necessary. Occupational therapists can advise on gadgetry for embroidery and craftwork; art therapists will guide creative artwork (or involve the local Art Society); most lending libraries can provide books and audio-tapes of books and music; organizations for the blind and partially-sighted will lend audio-cassette players and recorded newspapers, both national and local; and so forth. Don't overlook the use of computers and word-processors either, or the range of adaptations and computerized equipment available.

- Specialized gadgetry, and customized alterations or adaptations to off-the-shelf items, can be designed and made for individuals. In the UK, contact the nearest REMAP group for this. Composed of volunteers from local engineering and business firms, and an occupational therapist, they will produce anything from a wheelchair-mounted fishing-rod controllable by one hand, to a page-turner.

- Electric outdoor wheelchairs or shopping scooters give mobility to those whose walking is limited. A driving licence is not required for these in the UK, but make certain that the Stroke has the competence required: some cognitive impairments preclude the independent use of wheeled vehicles both indoors and outdoors (unilateral neglect, for instance).

- For Strokes who remain unable to reach such independence (and in the meantime) catalogue-shopping is one option. Sometimes local stores will deliver shopping orders and a few people (be careful and investigate their credentials) may operate a mobile service which will bring a range of clothes or shoes into a residential community or day centre.

- An extra walking-aid kept on the top landing is a great help for people with stairs. A grab-rail or handles fitted by the bannister, top and bottom, will keep a stick handy – hang one up at the bottom, collect the other at the top and vice versa. Rollators require space: fitted handrails on walls may provide an alternative means of support for getting about upstairs.

- Raising community awareness of the incidence and problems of stroke will help integration and assist any lobbying for improved or better facilities (including, perhaps, more rehabilitation units and/or specialist therapists).

TO SUMMARIZE

Responsibility, like caring, is an intricate balance between taking and giving, receiving and dispensing.

Delegation brings its own responsibility – for another's understanding of responsibility. It requires courage, discretion, and expert guidance.

Dependency feeds on sustained caregiving and the lack of responsibility. To rehabilitate people, subtle precautions need to be built in throughout the programme in order to prepare individuals for emotional independence as well as for physical independence. Certain Strokes find themselves ill-equipped in this respect, and carers can become trapped into giving extended and unnecessary support.

Stroke-survivors need to be weaned from dependence on formal rehabilitation programmes, from the rehabilitationists, from secure or institutional environments, and from 24-hour care.

Some carers need to be weaned from caretaking or caregiving.

Reintroduce enjoyment, the sense of belonging to the human race, acknowledge the fallibility of the system – any system! – reawaken a sense of adventure, hug each other occasionally, laugh together and don't be afraid to cry together (but not too often).

The ultimate goal must be the re-attainment of at least partial or shared personal autonomy, the sustainment of personal identity and the freedom to interact with confidence.

Surviving a stroke should reaffirm adulthood – and life.

The value of life is not the end of it, but the use we make of it.

(Molière)

REFERENCES

El-Din, D.J. (1991) *Iatrogenesis: Implications for Physical Therapy.* Proceedings of the World Confederation for Physical Therapists 11th International Congress, London, 28 July–2 August 1991, World Confederation of Physical Therapists, Book III, pp.1716–18.

Gilleard, C.J. (1991) Caring for people with dementia: some post-workshop reflections. *Generations, the Bulletin of the British Society of Gerontology,* **16**, 32–3.

Sarton, M. (1988) *After the Stroke: a journal,* The Women's Press, London.

PART FOUR
'Need-to-Know'

Essential Skills 13

The importance of solely therapeutic assistance and facilitation to enable a Stroke to accomplish every functional activity, however basic it may seem, has already been established, and the urgency of its application to neurological stressing was emphasized in the introduction to Chapter 10.

For a Stroke who is getting up for the first time, the process sets the pattern for optimal functional independence from the very beginning, even if it seems a forlorn hope at first.

Neglect, in the form of uninformed, too much, or total assistance for these familiar tasks, creates the dependent and traditionally disabled Stroke. Domestic routines form the primary rehabilitation structure, and without a consistent programme a Stroke may never regain the basic element of dynamic balance which enables the recovery of functional movement. The extra time and personnel that may be needed at this stage is more than compensated for as ability is quickly achieved (usually within a few days, but allow a couple of weeks for really severe strokes). The partner should be involved too. This can relieve pressure on staffing levels once the pattern is established, and help to create involvement and confident handling from the start.

For Strokes whose balance is severely impaired, the facilitation of automatic postural control takes precedence at all times. The Stroke has to concentrate on achieving and maintaining sitting and standing balance – protected and facilitated by a second helper if necessary – while the helper alongside (sitting to the S side) actually does all the washing and dressing for the Stroke, but following the same format each time in order to reinforce learning and continuity. As balance improves, the Stroke can be encouraged to take an increasingly active role.

Concentration on the task in hand, and the conscious control of posture and movement, very quickly result in exhaustion and the helper may need to take the decision either to complete the programme, or to let the Stroke relax on the bed for half-an-hour in a reflex-inhibiting position before resuming and completing the activity with active participation. Try to keep rooms comfortably warm and draught-free.

Colour-coding by sewing binding around apertures such as armholes, and markings to denote 'back' or 'right'/'left' of a garment, will help to identify the means of getting into them where there are figure-ground or spatial agnosias.

The first three sections refer to the first day post-stroke and/or to the very severely disabled, and are described in detail as a guide to ongoing practice. The degree of help required will vary according to individual need, as will the gradual withdrawal of assistance as abilities develop or change.

Work through the protocols steadily, in theory and then in practice – on a one-to-one basis with the Stroke until the format feels natural – then include other carers. Informed understanding of the importance of the procedure (enable or disable) ensures continuity, and the process rapidly becomes automatic and inbuilt into all future related activities. Stick to the format until the Stroke is confident – and able – enough to perform independently, then encourage more individual short cuts (but remain alert for adverse reactions).

13.1 Assisted washing and dressing
13.2 Assisted toileting
13.3 Assisted oral feeding
13.4 Getting on and off the floor

13.1 ASSISTED WASHING AND DRESSING

Identify, choose – with the help of the Stroke – and gather together all the necessary clothes, equipment and paraphernalia (including an extra towel for sitting on) first:

- a sturdy bedside table, adjusted to fit over the knees;
- two towels, preferably colour-coded – one for the face and top half, one for the lower half;
- two flannels, sponges, etc., colour-coded as above;
- one towel to sit on;
- talc, deodorant, etc.
- soap in non-slip soapdish (or on a moistened paper handtowel);
- washbowl – not too deep, half-filled with hand-hot clean water;
- teeth-cleaning (and fixing) necessities;
- hairbrush/comb;
- shaving equipment, etc.

Clear the bedding away from the Stroke, and place the 'sitting' towel on the edge of the bed alongside the S hip. Facilitate the Stroke to roll over to the S side and sit on the towel on the side of the bed, feet flat on a non-slip floor (adjust the bed height if necessary) slightly apart, and with weight distributed equally through the buttocks (check from behind). Assist the feet into slippers if the floor is chilly. Arrange the clothes to hand on the bed (to N side) ready to be put back on.

Working to the N side encourages trunk rotation with protraction of the S shoulder and stretching of the trunk musculature on the S side, and prevents the initiation of abnormal hypertonocity and reflexia.

This may be contrary to some traditional practice, but by now the reasoning should be obvious: try it! Turn from the waist to look to the left – as the right shoulder swings forward, the left shoulder twists back into retraction and the left elbow starts to flex.

Reaching to the N side to fetch articles will involve automatic postural adjustment for stability from the S side. It may also stimulate spontaneous S arm reaching or supporting activity (but don't ask for this, just watch).

Encourage and facilitate the natural use of both hands **if** there is some recovery of movement, but don't nag, and let the Stroke use the N hand if this is more appropriate and avoids distress and frustration. A smooth transition to rehabilitation is vital at this early stage, it is more important to give confidence, gain reciprocity and expedite the whole process as normally as possible, than it is to set inflexible rules (these can be absorbed later, in less personal circumstances).

The helper sits beside the Stroke on their S side, and is able to nudge or guide them back into balance whenever necessary, at the same time allowing sufficient free sway to give the Stroke the opportunity to feel the disturbance and start to correct it for themselves.

To maintain the Stroke's dignity, undressing, washing and dressing of the top half of the body can be completed before starting on the lower half.

TOP HALF

The table is positioned over the knees, but with enough space between abdomen and edge to allow leaning forwards (otherwise movement is curtailed). Place the bowl centrally and wash things to the N side, ready for use by the N hand, with the face towel across the knees. The helper has to be fairly ambidextrous in order to reach across for items with their 'outside' hand, when this is necessary.

Washing necessitates taking off nightwear, easier to do by pulling over the head (keep pyjama tops buttoned if they are roomy enough), a very good balance exercise!

Trunk stability requires dynamic coordination between flexors and extensors – the secret lies in not rushing the process, and encouraging the Stroke to lean slightly forwards, bending their head down as the clothing is grasped behind the neck in their active hand and gently pulled up and forwards until clear. The garment can then be pulled free from the S arm by the N hand, which can then gently shake or fiddle itself free from the remaining sleeve (the sleeve pressed against the thigh will fix it while the N arm is freed, better than using teeth!). A non-functional (thus far) S arm should be supported: forearm and elbow on the table if flaccid, on pillows alongside on the bed if tending towards hyper-reflexia (or the table will get swept clear!).

Then begin washing: face cloth into water and squeezed out, rubbed over soap (if used on the face) and face and neck cleansed. Rinse and towel dry. Repeat for whole top half of body – including under arms, under breasts and back. Helper may need to assist the attempt to get into the S armpit (perhaps merely by lifting the S arm gently away from the body) and under heavy breasts (again, gently lift away from the body) and to completely wash and dry the back. Ensure skin is thoroughly dried, and skin folds and crevices dusted with talc for ongoing comfort. Final rinse and squeeze for face flannel/sponge, and set it aside (easily overlooked in all the excitement). Move table aside and help collect garments, one at a time and in order, for dressing.

Getting into articles of clothing, and in the correct order, may need prompting if there is agnosia, dyspraxia or confusion caused by an inability to use or coordinate one set of limbs with the other.

Women are disadvantaged at this point: bras can be complex. There are several options:

- fasten it up at the front first (or get a front-fastening bra); this is difficult anyway – how to keep a hold on the S side long enough to fasten it without it catapulting away (clamping the S arm to the body sets up the abnormal reflex patterns of adduction, flexion and medial rotation) – then pull the bra around until the cups are in place, and struggle into straps;
- replace the fastening with similarly broad elastic, stretchy enough to allow the bra to be pulled on over the head and down to the waist, then the arms can be eased into the straps and the lot shrugged up into place;
- wear a bra-slip and put it on as above; the skirt can be chopped off to knicker length (or shorter) for wearing with trousers.

For tops and dresses, the N hand helps the S arm into its sleeve, then pushes its own way into its own sleeve, working the sleeves up as high as possible above the elbow. The back of the garment is collected up from bottom edge to neck, the neck opening pulled backwards over the lowered head and the whole lot pulled downwards into place, back, sides and front.

Long-sleeved garments can be laid across the lap, back uppermost and sleeves dangling between or beside the knees with the bottom edge opened ready to dive into. The S arm is then lowered down into the appropriate sleeve, followed by the N arm into its sleeve, working the fabric up the arm against the knee and thigh. Leaning to reach forwards in this way aborts the underlying extensor patterns of hyper-reflexia which disrupt normal dynamic postural control.

Shirts and cardigans can remain buttoned or zipped up if loose enough, and pulled on in the same way until dynamic balance is regained. This prevents the need to struggle into a sleeve behind the back which often triggers hyper-reflexia, and also maintains concentration on the basic issue of balance control undistracted by frustration with buttoning. (Buttoning skills can be developed once the Stroke is coping confidently with balance control.)

Dresses and skirts are simpler to don if pulled over the head and shoulders and worked down to the waist.

LOWER HALF

Lower garments are wriggled down to the thighs and clear of the bed, which necessitates weight-transference from side to side (assisted at first, perhaps, by a second helper supporting under the buttocks from behind and gently initiating the rocking movement). The second towel can then be draped discreetly across the lap for modesty if top garments are short.

Free the feet from slippers and the legs from pyjamas one at a time, N leg first (this puts weight through the S side and inhibits reflex activity). Leaning forward combined with reaching is part of this manoeuvre – the helper is there to control it, their nearside arm behind the Stroke and their outside arm free to intervene in front where necessary.

Raise the bed until the Stroke can perch securely nearer the edge, with thighs slanting downwards and feet appropriately re-adjusted. Bring the table to centre front again, just over knees (and a fresh bowl of water if it is now too cool or scummy). Use second flannel and towel to wash and dry personal areas and private parts. Assist the Stroke to lift each thigh just enough to reinforce weight transference to their other side to enable cleansing, drying and taking of the inner groin area and underneath, each side (another excellent natural balance exercise – try it!).

Move the table aside to deal with lower legs and feet. If reaching down this far is inadvisable, introduce sitting with one leg crossed over the other, and start with the S leg first – hooked over and supported on the N knee (unless obesity or arthritis renders this impossible, in which case try the S leg hooked over the helper's nearside knee, or support the foot on a low footstool). The helper may need to hold the S leg in place at first, and to help the changeover.

Crossing the N leg over the S leg is often more of an ordeal than would be expected, but persevere (insist, even) this first time. Sitting without support from the N leg and foot brings all the automatic postural adaptation of trunk musculature into action and produces probably the first instinctive supporting reactions in the S leg and foot. This is a particularly important stage when working with potential 'pushers' and Strokes with marked sensory loss – preventing the onset of compulsive weight-bearing on the N side.

If standing is possible at this stage (it should be, unless the balance reactions are totally chaotic), then this is an ideal time to initiate and practise rising from a sitting position (using the method outlined in Chapter 10). The helper, now in front and to the S side, allows the Stroke to come fully upright, and continues to support as necessary with nearside arm and knees while facilitating the washing, drying and powdering of the buttocks with the free hand. If the Stroke is very collapsible, a second helper may be needed for the actual washing and drying. Sitting down again (controlled relaxation from standing, remember) may be necessary during this procedure, for everyone's sake! Every change in position reinforces control of the CoG in relation to the BoS, so repetition progresses independence.

If standing cannot be achieved successfully, then side-rolling (from sitting) to half-lying on the S side enables this bit of the process to be carried out with the N hand. Return the Stroke to the sitting position.

For dressing the lower half, take one leg and clothe it completely before starting on the other. This may not seem normal, but it serves to give sufficient time in one position for all the dynamic balance reactions associated with that position to begin to re-establish themselves (and also prevents bare or stockinged feet slipping about on the floor). As soon as the Stroke is dynamically safe, the more usual pre-stroke methods can be resumed, subject of course to precautionary reflex-inhibiting postures.

Clothe the S leg first, leg over knee as for washing.

If an elasticated support stocking is worn, this is the time to pull it on. A gadget like a metal tubular scaffolding is sometimes supplied, but otherwise the helper needs to grasp the stocking firmly at the top using both hands (thumbs inside) and scrabble down to the toe collecting it all together with fingers and thumbs. Then, leaning across the Stroke so that body pressure is bearing down on the S knee (still crossed over the N knee), place the toe aperture – with thumbs inside to keep it open – over the toes and pull on and up steadily (ensuring S knee stays flexed), unravelling the stocking as it is applied to the leg. Keep a good grip on it and control the stretch appropriately, and ease your own body away from the S knee to complete the procedure up the S thigh if a full-length garment is used. Smooth out little wrinkles by 'massaging' over the garment. This is a very quick and simple method and much easier than it looks. So if the stocking has twisted or gone awry altogether, peel it off and start again. The final adjustments at the top of the thigh can be made later, when all the lower garments are pulled up into place.

Then – or otherwise – start with the underpants, retrieved by the Stroke with their active hand, shaken out with front and back identified and held at the top band on the side which matches the N side. The dangling leg opening is then looped over the S foot and worked up to the knee. Then the sock or ordinary stocking, then the trouser leg (if trousers are being worn) and finally the shoe.

The S leg is replaced, foot firmly on the floor (and shod to increase stability), and then the N foot can be helped – in the same order – into its respective openings. This takes great courage the first time, as both the N leg and N hand are occupied functionally and cannot be utilized for support (very therapeutic).

The N side of lower garments are held in the N hand, underpants first, and lowered for easier access to just below the S knee again. Sometimes it is simpler to reach behind and under the N leg so that the N foot can just be 'stepped' backwards into the aperture. Trouser leg next, and garments pulled right up the thighs.

If standing is achievable, facilitate the rise from sitting, and control balance in standing while the clothing is pulled up with the N hand and adjusted for comfort. As in sitting with the N leg across the S knee, using the N hand functionally while standing reinforces symmetrical weight-bearing and prevents it being used as a prop. Habitual use of the N arm as an extra leg creates the traditional disabilities and denies its normal usage.

The helper can support, as before, to maintain equilibrium with appropriate nudges and practical assistance. If standing is not possible, the Stroke remains sitting and leans sideways to hitch up the garments on one side and repeats the performance from side to side until everything is comfortably in place (this reinforces dynamic weight transference). Finally the N leg is crossed over the S knee so that both sock and shoe can be pulled on.

Outer garments such as cardigans, jackets, anoraks and overcoats present difficulty and the ensuing struggle can disrupt all the carefully-nurtured normality achieved in the dressing routine. Avoid this by assisting the S arm in first, but keep the garment 'off-the-shoulder' and low across the back so that the N arm can plunge easily into the other sleeve at about waist level. Then the top of the coat can be assisted up into place over the shoulders with a natural bilateral shrugging action.

These procedures for washing and dressing indicate the manner in which assistance and facilitation interlink to promote and enable carry-over into ongoing functional activity. The same thoughtful approach must be incorporated into all the activities of daily living, night and day, until the Stroke is coping with minimal – or no – assistance. Strokes will regain independence surprisingly fast in this way, except for the unfortunate few with severe CNS damage who will be enabled to progress to their optimal potential but may continue to require help with certain activities.

Occupational therapists will advise on bath aids and devise individual ways and means for having a bath.

A shower is useful. If necessary, a plastic 'patio' chair can be brought in to sit on, its legs stabilized on a non-slip mat or a wet towel.

If a shower isn't available, a **secure board across the bath** is easy to transfer on to before swinging the legs over the edge and into the bath: sitting on this and using a shower-hose attachment from the taps is an alternative.

Little bath stools, often supplied with the bath-board to give a second lower seat prior to actually sitting down in the bath itself, require real strength and agility and can trigger all the abnormal reflexia, and therefore are not recommended for general use (try it – extensor patterns come into action as the shoulders take the weight of the body, and grazes across the back from the edge of the bath-board are common as the trunk slithers down to sit on the stool).

Non-slip mats in the bath or shower cubicle prevent falls and slithering – a wet towel works but is not so stable.

Wet and/or soapy skin is slippery, so it can be helpful if the Stroke wears clean underpants to bath in (roomy enough to be able to wash inside them): this enables a firm hold for helpers to assist manoeuvring.

13.2 ASSISTED TOILETING

This precedes washing and dressing at the beginning of the day, but for many people working with the stroke-disabled the need to assist a Stroke to the lavatory usually occurs during other episodes of treatment. It is part of everyday functional activity and as such must be clearly recognized as continuing therapy. Notice the emphasis on 'assist' – to 'get' an individual to the loo denies the possibility of independence.

The transfer on to a commode, or into a wheelchair (S foot on footplate!) for a journey to a suitable toilet and then on to the lavatory, must be facilitated as described in Chapter 10. If it is a matter of urgency, clothing can be pulled clear during the 'swivel' (helpers' arms supporting body while hands arrange garments) so that on being re-seated on to the commode/lavatory no further time need be wasted. Otherwise use the occasion to practise transfers and sitting-to-standing-to-sitting – it also helps bladder re-training ('hang on while...'). The Stroke sits on the toilet seat to complete the transfer, then comes up to standing while clothing is worked clear, and then is allowed to sit down for emptying. This is easier for the helper, too.

Whenever possible allow men to stand (discreetly supporting and maintaining balance from behind) to urinate. Much more natural, and easier than manhandling in the sitting position (particularly with heavy people).

Women should be encouraged to wipe themselves (this can be done from the front) after passing urine.

Cleaning involves leaning forwards and maintaining equilibrium while twisting to reach behind. Facilitate balance and be prepared to hand over the appropriate tissue and to take over if necessary.

Facilitate standing again (rescuing slipping garments too). Pulling up underpants and adjusting clothing afterwards can be done by the Stroke, with some assistance if required. It's unfair to insist on active participation beforehand, as time may be at a premium then!

Then make time for handwashing. Encourage the Stroke to turn taps, test the temperature, use soap and find towels (and to pull the plug out afterwards).

13.3 ASSISTED ORAL FEEDING

Practise on a colleague with unimpaired swallowing – and be practised on – until the procedure can be safely, skilfully and comfortably accomplished.

Never attempt to give a drink or food to anyone who is not fully conscious and aware that liquid or more solid matter is being offered.

Keep paper tissues or soft clean cloths to hand, and make sure that help from professional or emergency services is within call.

Be prepared to clear out obstructing food from the mouth fast if choking is indicated, and go into the appropriate first-aid routine.

The following method applies to Strokes who have been assessed by specialist professionals (who will advise on the appropriate texture or type of nourishment to be offered, and on any specific procedure to adhere to) and who are fully aware and co-operating, but who require maximum assistance – the degree of help actually needed must be judged accordingly at each stage of each meal.

The helper sits beside, but higher than, the Stroke (on the arm of the chair for instance), nearside arm behind the neck to lightly cradle the person's head in the crook of the elbow with hand gently curved round the facial contour at jaw level – thumb against the temporomandibular joint, index finger under nose above upper lip (without obstructing the nostrils!), middle finger under lower lip and other fingers supporting just under the point of the jaw (with no pressure against the throat) – so that the head is upright, but can be gently tilted forwards or backwards, and lip and jaw closure can be facilitated.

For liquids, small sips from a teaspoon are recommended to start with.

Small spoonfuls (about a third of a teaspoonful) of food are presented with the other hand and need to be guided into the lips and on to the tongue, and lip closure facilitated.

Keep head level – forwards, the food will fall out; if it is backwards, there is a danger of it going straight back and into the airway.

Put the spoon down and facilitate the chewing of solid matter with small-range up and down jaw movement if necessary, and/or verbal prompting.

When a swallow is indicated, tilt the head slightly downwards and give firm pressure into the musculature under the jaw to stimulate the extrinsic tongue muscles, and massage downwards with the thumb and fingers of the other hand to each side of the trachea (without compressing it) with gentle static pressure to the hyoid bone.

As chewing and swallowing become easier, progress to more normal mouthfuls. For liquids, progress to sipping from a cup, facilitating normal holding of the cup or spoon as well until the Stroke is competent enough to cope more independently. Supervision is necessary for a considerable period after this stage is reached; choking is an ongoing and all-too-frequent hazard for dysarthric Strokes.

Dysphagic Strokes have impairment of all the stages of swallowing and will probably require nasogastric tube-feeding at first: severe cases may need to continue with this. The decision to start oral feeding should be taken with the speech and language therapist, and the efficiency of the swallowing mechanism can be further assessed by videofluoroscopy.

13.4 GETTING ON AND OFF THE FLOOR

Even the most carefully orchestrated activities do not prevent an occasional fall – accidents can and do happen. Obviously it is better to control and practise the getting-up procedure as soon as possible so that the process is less alarming when it occurs unplanned! As with all assisted activity, practise it (and be practised on) first with able colleagues so that the basic moves are already well-learned.

GETTING DOWN

In order to get up from the floor, it is necessary to first get down on to the floor – in itself quite an anxious undertaking, especially for the older Strokes. It requires plenty of time, space and reassurance:

1. Start with the Stroke sitting on the edge of the lowest chair or plinth available, with a stool or firm armless chair placed in front of the knees within comfortable reach. Some Strokes prefer to perch sideways, turned to the N side, and to slide down on to the S knee from this position.
2. Encourage reaching forwards to lean on this second seat, in the centre if the Stroke is only using one hand, or by grasping the sides with both hands.
3. The Stroke will be expected to take bodyweight on to the N hand/forearm – or both hands if the S arm is safely functional – while sliding the S foot far enough back (under the seat being sat on), so that weight can then be transferred down on to the S knee which by this time should be down on the floor. Facilitate these actions by guiding the foot and knee into position and supporting the S-shoulder and some bodyweight if necessary.
4. When this position is achieved, some further support may be needed while the Stroke slides the N leg down into kneeling.
5. The N arm is then placed down to the floor on the N side so that with a gentle swing of the hips to the N side 'side-sitting' can be accomplished – on the floor.
6. From here to forearm support and then to side-lying, on the N side.

GETTING UP

If the Stroke has fallen, then the priority must be to assess for acute injury, and the appropriate first-aid or emergency routine instituted if injuries are suspected.

Otherwise the first stage is to help the Stroke into a more comfortable position (with a pillow or cushion under the head if possible), while the environment is checked and furniture rearranged for the next stage. Encourage the Stroke to assess this also, and reassure throughout. Remember that all activity is part of the rehabilitation scheme, and any manoeuvre is just another opportunity for functional re-education.

Sit down on the floor with the Stroke before starting, and work alongside whenever possible to reinforce the self-help concept. Only resort to a total take-over if the individual is unable to cooperate at all.

To begin with, the Stroke needs to roll into side-lying on the N side, raise up to take weight on to the N forearm (or hand), and then bottom-shunt sideways to lean against a stable object – a low chair or stool (or anything else convenient like the bottom step of a staircase or the lavatory with lid down, for instance). Both knees should remain flexed and side-sitting maintained. Short rests may be needed during or after each stage. If help is required, it should be unobtrusive and simple – a little hoist from the back of the waistband, perhaps, for each lift-and-shunt across the intervening space, assistance to keep the S knee flexed, or to fetch the furniture alongside to lean on if the Stroke is tiring.

Still in side-sitting, the Stroke finishes alongside the chosen piece of furniture. The N arm is then lifted to self-support on the seat and the Stroke comes up to kneeling (still N-side towards), and then one foot (whichever feels most secure) is brought up into place (flat on the ground) for the final push-up and bottom-swing to sit on the seat.

Some individuals have their own strong ideas regarding the best way to proceed: go along with it, try it all ways, be pragmatic. One man returned from his first (well-rehearsed) visit home and told how he had fallen while attempting to get from the wheelchair into a rocking-chair in the kitchen (this transfer had not been rehearsed!). 'Stupid fool,' his wife commented, as staff worried around him for signs of damage. 'You got him up the way we showed you?' asked the therapist. 'No – she just sat there,' complained the Stroke. He was anosognosic as a result of the stroke ('He's always been bloody-minded,' said his wife) and had argued with her until she gave up on him, fetched herself an ordinary chair and sat on it, arms folded. Furious, he then crawled up her, so to speak, and hauled himself up to his feet again, 'and swearing. He does better when he's angry', she explained, catching his eye, and they both laughed. This method could be added to the list for future reference!

It's not what you do, it's the way that you do it that matters.

(Laidler)

Resource materials 14

These guidelines are collected from the text, as are the picture charts, for use as *aides-mémoire*.

14.1 PROFESSIONAL GUIDELINES

Normal movement is in relation to gravity: CoG is the Centre of Gravity; BoS is the Base of Support, i.e. that which supports the body against gravity – feet, thighs, chair etc. A simple equation for dynamic balance and functional movement is:

$$\frac{CoG}{BoS} \ = \ \text{stability}$$

$$CoG - BoS \ = \ \text{instability}$$

CoG:BoS (controlled movement of CoG relative to BoS)
$$= \text{mobility} + \text{stability}$$
$$= \text{functional movement}$$

Dynamic postural control anticipates and allows freedom of peripheral limb movement.

Normal movement generates normal movement – it opens and re-opens pathways, and introduces natural control of inhibition and excitation. So to facilitate normal movement is to launch an ongoing process towards normality.

Gross patterns of movement precede fragmented components of movement.

Familiar and task- and context-specific actions can prompt a natural and spontaneous follow-through, and can also re-lay the rules to assist response selection for 'carry-over' into other activities.

Physiological stressing – repetition over a period of time – reinforces plastic adaptation and can therefore enable **and** disable people.

Controlled environmental factors help to ensure stability and continuity for the rehabilitation process.

14.2 PRACTICAL GUIDELINES

Cultivate heightened awareness of own and others' normal motor behaviour, and relate it to individual Strokes for problem-solving.

Always start with something the Stroke can achieve easily, and return to it if stuck (or depressed).

Coordinate therapy sessions. If standing balance has just been achieved in the physiotherapy department, then incorporate it into occupational therapy activity; if naming objects or the use of Amer-Ind is on the agenda in speech therapy, then incorporate this into the other therapies; if the Stroke has been standing for a while in OT, then it may be better to begin with sitting activities in the ensuing session to prevent fatigue.
   A little and often is a better way to build stamina and sustain carry-over into daily activity. Even changing weight-bearing positions reinforces the natural dynamics of postural adjustments.

Mime, gesture, repeat, rephrase, facilitate or physically prompt, and allow time for slow synapsing when responses are unforthcoming or unexpected. If there is still confusion, analyse the cause. If stuck, go on to something else before frustration sets in.

Monitor entire body activity and utilize mass movement synergies, even during explicit limb work. It is not normal for any part of the body to work in isolation.

Inhibit all stereotyped abnormal reflexia. Weight-bearing through proximal joints stimulates natural inhibitory systems, normal movement generates normal movement (and vice versa). This applies **24 hours a day**, including mealtimes, speech therapy sessions, doctor's rounds and in transit between therapies in the care of a porter – except possibly in dire emergencies like earthquake, fire or cardiac arrest.

Passive movements are not rehabilitative. If the Stroke is unconscious, limbs should be moved in large normal patterns not in their component parts, and rolling and turning should be carried out to replicate the natural movement incorporating trunk rotation.

Static poses are unproductive; it is the control of dynamic movement that is needed to restore normal functional activity.

Don't make a 'patient sandwich' – work and intervene from one side only (the S side wherever possible) and limit physical and verbal contact to just one source to maintain concentration and avoid distraction and confusion, until distraction is deliberately introduced as a therapeutic strategy to further progress.

Facilitate – evaluate. Be pragmatic – if it works, do it; if it doesn't, don't! (Try again later if it still seems potentially useful.) This applies to special techniques, too. Facilitation (clueing and prompting through handling) of normal movement at all times is the primary objective. An empirical approach requires objective evaluation.

Ensure that your own CoG doesn't fall outside your own BoS by keeping your feet apart in standing, and sit down whenever possible to utilize your own bodyweight and free hands for more sophisticated control (and to conserve your energy). A Stroke is entitled to balance problems, but a helper isn't! Avoid stressing the spinal column – back problems can be irreversible.

Make and maintain contact with appropriately-specializing professionals – and seek guidance and/or cross-refer for problem-solving, or for help in recognizing problems – throughout.

14.3 GENERAL MEMO FOR CARERS

All care is based on the prevention of spasticity, the avoidance of abnormal reflex patterns and the guidance of only normal movement, by careful handling and assistance.

- **put picture charts over beds**
  To remind other carers.
- **struggling increases problems**
  Don't ask the Stroke to try harder! Avoid effort, frustration, 'monkey-poles' and squeezing a handball.
- **avoid painful shoulder**
  No arm movements unless the **whole** shoulder area (including the shoulderblade) is relaxed and supple. Never lift the Stroke under the stroke arm, or pull it.
- **prevent dislocation**
  By supporting forearm and hand forwards, with natural weight through the elbow.
- **hands together**
  Linked or clasped while the Stroke is moving about, to prevent over-use of the non-stroke hand until normal balance is under control.
- **walking can wait**
  Until dynamic balance in standing and stepping is under control. 'Being walked' before this teaches dependency on other people, and delays recovery.
- **all walking must be good walking**
  With assistance where needed. After a stroke this may require:

helper(s)	supporting one or both sides, hands and arms supported in downthrust position (see handling chart 14.5).
a rollator	used to stimulate supportive action in the hand and arm; never use a Zimmer-type frame.
a walking stick	when the Stroke can walk a few steps unaided.
a quadrupod	if the Stroke is frail, poorsighted or clumsy.

- **walking is leaving one leg behind**
  Always step 'best foot forwards' first, and each step must be in front of the other foot (not merely up to it). Encourage turning to the hemiplegic side, and walking backwards, too.
- **'look behind you!'**
  In standing, and before sitting down, to improve balance reactions and mobility – and to find the chair!
- **quality not quantity**
  It's not what you do but the way that you do it that matters!

14.4 POSITIONING CHARTS

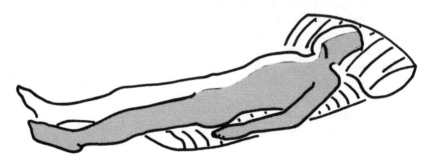

(a) Supported supine lying.

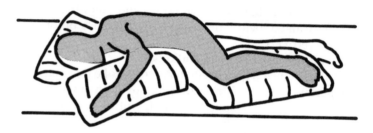

(b) Lying on the N side.

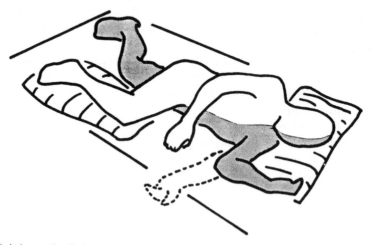

(c) Lying on the S side.

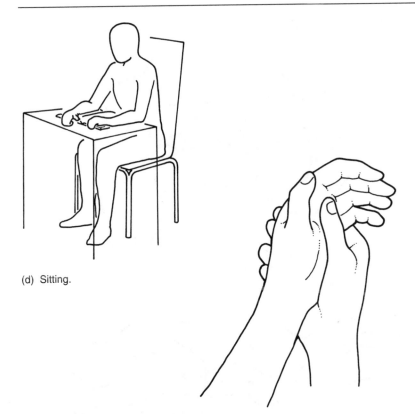

(d) Sitting.

(e) Supporting the S hand.

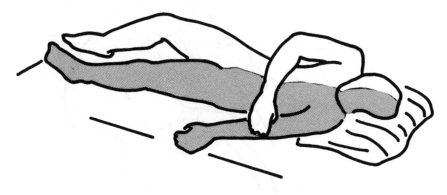

(f) Rolling to the S side.

14.5 HANDLING CHARTS

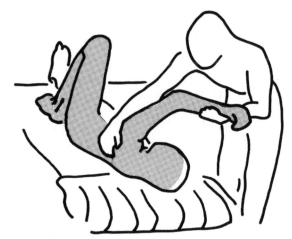

(a) Rolling to the N side.

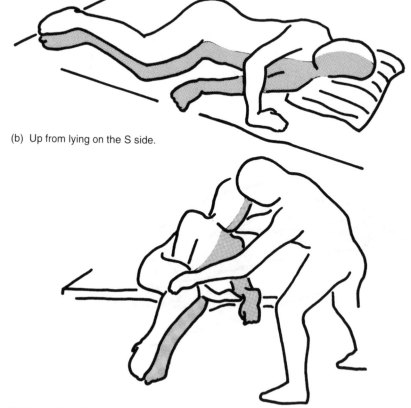

(b) Up from lying on the S side.

(c) Up to sit on the side of the bed.

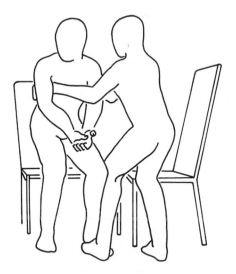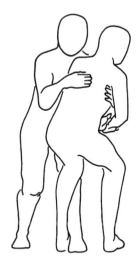

(d) The swivel transfer.

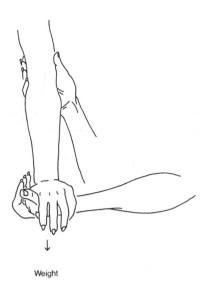

Weight

(f) Thumb-to-thumb S hand support.

14.6 AMER-IND GESTURES

Some of the more familiar gestural signs from this augmentative communication system.

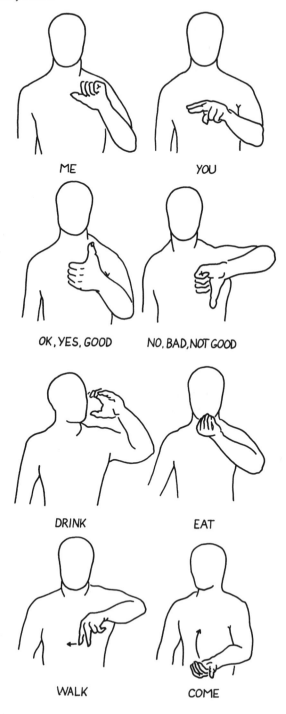

ME   YOU

OK, YES, GOOD   NO, BAD, NOT GOOD

DRINK   EAT

WALK   COME

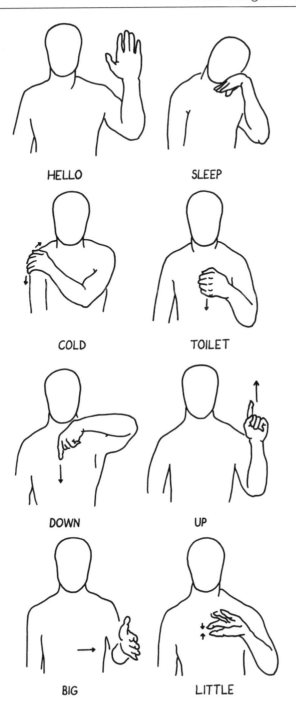

HELLO

SLEEP

COLD

TOILET

DOWN

UP

BIG

LITTLE

Postscript

THE OBJECTIVE OF ALL
DEDICATED COMPANY EMPLOYEES
SHOULD BE TO ANALYSE THOROUGHLY
ALL SITUATIONS, ANTICIPATE ALL
PROBLEMS PRIOR TO THEIR
OCCURRENCE, HAVE ANSWERS FOR
THESE PROBLEMS, AND MOVE
SWIFTLY TO SOLVE THESE PROBLEMS
WHEN CALLED UPON.
HOWEVER
WHEN YOU ARE UP TO YOUR ARSE
IN ALLIGATORS,
IT IS DIFFICULT TO REMEMBER
THAT YOUR INITIAL OBJECTIVE
WAS TO DRAIN THE SWAMP

Memo found pinned to the wall in
a social worker's office.

But please try!

Collected quotations

From the text and from the author's personal collection.

> He lik'd those literary cooks
> Who skim the cream of others' books;
> And ruin half an author's graces
> By plucking bon-mots from their places.
> (Hannah More, 1745–1833, *Florio*)

> Action is meaningless without the substratum of the idea.
> (Nick Miller, *Dyspraxia and its Management*)

> Little strokes fell great oaks . . .
> (Benjamin Franklin, 1706–1790)

> The important thing is to add life to years, not years to life.
> (Lord Amulree, doyen of geriatric medicine)

> A University should be a place of light, of liberty, and of learning.
> (Benjamin Disraeli, 1804–1881, a speech in the House of Commons
> 1873 – and so should a rehabilitation department!)

> 'There are strings,' said Mr Tappertit, 'in the human heart that had
> better not be wibrated.'
> (Charles Dickens, 1812–1870, *Barnaby Rudge*)

> The nervous system regulates and integrates the systems of the body
> and it provides for the behaviour and intellectual attainments of
> man.
> (Murray Llewellyn Barr, 1979)

> What we have to learn to do, we learn by doing.
> (Aristotle, 384–322 BC)

Habit is the enormous flywheel of society, its most precious conservative agent.

(William James, 1842–1910, *Psychology* 1)

Man is one chain of excitation surrounded by a wall of inhibition.

(Charles Scott Sherrington, 1857–1952)

When you are down, everything falls on you.

(Sylvia Townsend Warner, *The Fatal Law of Gravity*)

We think in generalities, but we live in detail.

(Alfred North Whitehead, 1861–1947)

... that to live is to change, and to be perfect is to have changed often.

(Cardinal Newman, 1801–1890)

If a man will begin with certainties, he shall end in doubts, but if he will be content to begin with doubts, he shall end in certainties.

(Francis Bacon, 1561–1626, *The Advancement of Learning*)

also

They are ill discoverers that think there is no land, when they can see nothing but sea.

There are no known facts, merely the current theory of the day.

(Carl Popper, paraphrased by Professor Jack Howell)

The brain knows nothing of muscles, only of movement.

(FMR Walshe, 1923)

Go not forth hastily to strive, lest thou know not what to do in the end thereof.

(Old Testament, Book of Proverbs 23:35)

Life is the art of drawing sufficient conclusions from insufficient premises.

(Samuel Butler, 1835–1902, *Note-books, Life*)

'I am a lone lorn creetur', were Mrs Gummidge's words ... 'and everythink goes contrairy with me.'

(Charles Dickens, 1812–1870, *David Copperfield*)

If the brain were so simple that we could understand it, we would be so simple that we couldn't.

(Emerson Pugh, 1977)

He that hath no rule over his own spirit is like a city that is broken down, and without walls.

(Old Testament, Book of Proverbs 25:28)

Go through what is comprehensible and you conclude that only the incomprehensible gives any light.

(Saul Bellow, 1915–, *Herzog*)

Dogma does not mean absence of thought, but the end of thought.

(G.K. Chesterton, 1874–1936)

It is better to understand little than to misunderstand a lot.

(Anatole France, 1844–1924)

For verily the tribe is all, and we are nothing singly save as parts of it.

(James Thomson, 1834–1882)

Nine-tenths of wisdom is being wise in time.

(Theodore Roosevelt, 1858–1919)

Boast not thyself of tomorrow, for thou knowest not what a day may bring forth.

(Old Testament, Book of Proverbs 27:1)

In nature there are neither rewards nor punishments – there are consequences.

(Robert Ingersoll, 1833–1899, *Lectures & Essays*)

In the field of observation, chance favours only the prepared minds.

(Louis Pasteur, 1822–1895)

Look to the future with vigour and not with fondness on the past.

(Geoffrey Kidd, 1988)

The most melancholy of human reflections, perhaps, is that, on the whole, it is a question whether the benevolence of mankind does most good or harm.

(Walter Bagehot, 1826–1877, *Physics and Politics*)

The value of life is not the end of it, but the use we make of it.

(Molière, 1622–1673)

Age is mostly a matter of mind: if you don't mind, it doesn't matter.

(anon.)

The key to longevity is to keep breathing.

(Sophie Tucker)

What divides men is less a difference in ideas than a likeness in pretensions.

(Pierre-Jean de Beranger, 1780–1857)

Life is one long process of getting tired.

(Samuel Butler, 1835–1902, *Note-books, Life*)

The feeling of sleepiness when you are not in bed, and can't get there, is the meanest feeling in the world.

(E.W. Howe, *Country Town Sayings*)

Have the courage to live – anyone can die.

(Robert Cody)

Experience is the name every one gives to their mistakes.

(Oscar Wilde, 1854–1900, *Lady Windermere's Fan*)

also

'The English country gentleman galloping after a fox – the unspeakable in full pursuit of the uneatable.'

(*A Woman of No Importance*)

also

There is no sin except stupidity.

(*The Critic as Artist, Part 2*)

Cooking? Nothing to it – if it's brown it's done: if it's black it's buggered.

(anon.)

Any stigma will do to beat a dogma.

(Philip Guedalla, 1889–1944)

A clash of doctrines is not a disaster – it is an opportunity.

(Alfred North Whitehead, 1861–1947)

When people's ill, they come to I,
I physicks, bleeds and sweats 'em.
Sometimes they live, sometimes they die.
What's that to I? I 'lets 'em'!

(Dr John Lettsom, 1744–1815)

Around, around the sun we go:
the moon goes round the earth.
We do not die of death:
we die of vertigo

(Archibald MacLeish, 1892–)

An Expert is someone who comes from somewhere else – with slides.

(source unknown)

An expert is one who knows more and more about less and less.

(Nicholas Butler, 1862–1947)

It isn't for the dead I grieve,
it is for the living, whom the dead bereave.

(source unknown)

Genius is one per cent inspiration and ninety-nine per cent perspiration.

(Thomas Edison, 1847–1931)

Gift, like genius, I often think means only an infinite capacity for taking pains.

(Jane Hopkins, 1836–1904)

The art of medicine is to keep the patient occupied while the disease run its course.

(Voltaire, 1694–1778)

Time is the great physician.

(Benjamin Disraeli, 1804–1881, *Henrietta Temple*)

Wherever a doctor cannot do good, he must be kept from doing harm.

(Hippocrates, c. 460–347 BC)

also

The life so short, the craft so long to learn.

Look wise, say nothing, and grunt. Speech was given to conceal thought.

(Sir William Osler, 1849–1919)

also

Half of us are blind, few of us feel, and we are all deaf.

also

It is astonishing with how little reading a doctor can practise medicine, but it is not astonishing how badly he may do it.

also

Don't touch the patient – State first what you see.

To be engaged in opposing wrong affords but a slender guarantee for being right.

(William Ewart Gladstone, 1809–1898)

Mankind, when left to themselves, are unfit for their own government.

(George Washington, 1732–1799)

also

Liberty, when it begins to take root, is a plant of rapid growth.

Poverty is an anomaly to rich people. It is very difficult to make out why people who want dinner do not ring the bell.

(Walter Bagehot, 1826–1877, *Literary Studies*)

Politics – the art of making the inevitable appear to be a matter of wise human choice.

(Quentin Crisp, 1991)

The English are busy; they don't have time to be polite.

(Baron de Montesquieu, 1689–1755)

Marriage, Agnes, is not a joke.

(Molière, 1622–1673)

Three passions, simple but overwhelmingly strong, have governed my life: the longing for love, the search for knowledge, and unbearable pity for the suffering of mankind.

(Bertrand Russell, 1872–1970)

also

Every man, wherever he goes, is encompassed by a cloud of comfortable convictions which move with him like flies on a summer day.

Success is the postponement of failure.

(Graham Greene, 1904–1993)

A detour is the wrong way to the right place.

(source unknown)

Never trouble Trouble
'til Trouble troubles you.
It only doubles trouble,
And troubles others, too.

(anon.)

In baiting a mouse-trap with cheese, always leave room for the mouse.

('Saki' – the author Hugh Munro, 1870–1916, *The Square Egg*)

also

He's simply got the instinct for being unhappy highly developed.

(*Chronicles of Clovis, The Match-Maker*)

A woman without a man is like a fish without a bicycle.

(graffiti)

also

I wish I was what I was when I wished I was what I am now.

I'm breathless with work...

(my grandmother's elderly neighbour)

Withhold not good from them to whom it is due, when it is in the power of thine hand to do it.

(Old Testament, Book of Proverbs 3:13)

Good words without deeds are rushes and reeds.

(proverb, first referenced in 1659)

Beware of all enterprises that require fancy clothes.

(H.D. Thoreau, 1817–1862)

What is the use of running when we are not on the right road?

(German proverb)

You can fool too many of the people too much of the time.

(James Thurber, 1894–1961)

The hounds of obsolescence are nipping at our heels.

(Ruth Grant, 1991)

My life has been blessed throughout with wonderful people who have helped me to learn and grow. Their relentless hard work and love make the success of any book I work on theirs as well.

(Ken Hom, *East Meets West*)

The author and publisher would like to thank all the owners and controllers of copyright of the quotations sprinkled throughout the text and listed here. These have been collected over many years by the author, with their published source unrecorded (and in most instances not known). If the copyright owners would write to the publisher, the appropriate acknowledgements can be given in the next edition.

GLOSSARY

a- As a prefix, it indicates the total loss of that ability.

Afferent Pathways or signals passing towards a structure (the brain): usually relates to sensory input.

Agnosia Generic term indicating a failure to recognize certain familiar objects although the senses are intact: sensations without perception.

Agonists The muscles contracting to produce movement at a joint, the 'prime movers'.

Aides memoires Reminders.

Analogue A collection of corresponding facts.

Anomaly An irregularity, a deviation from the norm.

Anosodiaphoria Abnormal lack of concern about the situation.

Anosognosia Failure to recognize or understand one's own disability and therefore the inability to relate to it, or to remember strategies for dealing with it.

Antagonists Opposing muscle group which should be reciprocally innervated to relax in order to allow movement at a joint.

Aphagia Functional loss of the swallowing mechanisms.

Aphasia Inability to express oneself through speech and/or to comprehend the spoken word. Can apply to written language and to gestures and symbols too.

Apraxia Generic term for an inability to perform purposeful movements even though motor power, sensation and intellect may be unimpaired.

Articulatory loop A memory system that utilizes subvocal speech.

Asymmetrical tonic neck reflex Rotation of the head to one side elicits extension of the arm on that side, with flexion of the arm on the opposite side.

Ataxia Unco-ordinated movement, characterized by increased postural sway, lurching gait, clumsiness.

Atheroma Deposit on the lining of arteries.

Atherosclerosis Furring up of the linings of arterial walls.

Audit Systematic examination of data.

Auto-inhibition Self-induced, utilizing the natural inhibitory systems, as against mechanically-induced inhibition by the use of ice, inflatable splints, etc.

Autonomic system The part of the nervous system that controls the smooth muscle tissue for the visceral functions of the body.

Axial/proximal Central to, nearest to the centre of, the body.

Axon Neuronal fibril that transmits impulses to other neurons and effector organs.

Bilateral discrimination A test for equality of sensation at both points when the same stimulation is applied simultaneously to the same point on the S- and the N-limb.

Biofeedback Procedure that permits individuals to monitor their own physical or physiological processes or performance, to learn to control them.

Biogenesis Biological origins.

Biosocial Sociological factors determining or implicated in living or wellbeing.

BoS Base of Support.

CAT scan Computerized Axial Tomography.

Central executive CNS coordinating component. controlling functions and allocating resources during task processing. Breakdown in this area is thought to cause the problems seen in Alzheimer's disease.

CNS Central Nervous System.

Co-contraction Simultaneous contraction of all muscles around a joint preventing movement at that joint, as in spasticity.

CoG Centre of Gravity.

Cognition Knowledge, collection and perception of incoming signals for thought-processing and the organization of functional ability.

Consensus General agreement.

Concomitant Accompanying.

Connotation Implication, association.

Criteria Standards by which something can be judged.

CVA Cerebral Vascular Accident, resulting in a stroke.

Demographic Pertaining to population statistics.

Dendrite The neuronal tendril that receives incoming signals.

Doctrine Accepted teachings or principles.

Dogma Theory or doctrine asserted on authority without supporting evidence.

DREZ Dorsal Root Entry Zone.

dys- As a prefix denotes a partial loss of that ability.

Dysarthria Difficulty in articulation, eating and drinking due to weakness of the muscles of the face, mouth and throat.

Dysfunction Disordered functioning.

Dysphagia Impoverished swallowing mechanism.

Dysphasia Disorder of language: impaired expression and comprehension of speech and/or written language, gestures and symbols.

Dyspraxia Disorder in functional ability: confused performance of purposeful movements even though motor power, sensation and intellect may be unimpaired.

Efferent Pathways or signals travelling away from the brain: usually motor output.

Emboli Mobile debris in the arteries.

Emotionalism Inappropriate or excessive crying or laughing; emotional lability.

Engram A lasting mark or trace, the pattern of effect of a stimulation remaining in nervous tissue.

Episodic memory Autobiographical, personal record of events.

eu- The opposite of dys-, a combining form meaning well, easily or good.

Eutrophic Enhancing or recovering protein synthesis (nutrition) in tissues.

Excretion The expelling of waste matter, faeces.

Exogenous External to the central system.

Facilitate Make easier.

Facilitation Handling which prompts, assists and guides normal movements.

Feedback System by which information on the result of a process or activity modifies its further development.

Fusimotor Motor nerve fibres (of gamma motoneurons) that innervate intrafusal fibres of the muscle spindle.

GABA Gamma-AminoButyric Acid, an inhibitory neurotransmitter.

Ganglion Cluster of nerve cell bodies located outside the CNS.

Generic Pertaining to a group or species.

Glitch A sudden irregularity, a malfunction.

Glycolytic Muscle fibre metabolism converting glucose to lactate for energy.

Habituation Gradual adaptation to a stimulus or to the environment.

Hemianopia Defective vision or blindness in half of the visual field of one or both eyes.

Hemiplegia Deficiency of movement on one side of the body.

Heuristic A problem-solving technique that proceeds by trial and error, or one that furthers progress but is otherwise unproved or unjustified.

Holistic Relating to organic and functional relations between parts and a whole; entire.

Homeostasis The body's physico-chemical equilibrium.

Homogeneous Consisting or composed of similar elements or ingredients, of a uniform quality throughout.

Homogenous Having a similarity of structure because of descent from a common ancestor.

Homonymous hemianopia Hemianopia affecting the right halves or the left halves of the visual fields of both eyes, i.e. the side affected by the stroke.

Hyper-reflexia Uninhibited or poorly-controlled spinal reflex activity.

Hypertension High blood pressure.

Hypertonicity Increased muscle tone.

Hypotonicity Apparent weakness of muscle tissue due to reduced tone.

Iatrogenesis Any adverse mental or physical condition resulting from treatment.

Indirect exercise Planned exercising for the N-side of the body which prompts reciprocal automatic responses on the S-side.

Infarction Obstructed circulation, usually due to a thrombus or embolus, resulting in an area of coagulation necrosis.

Inhibition Arrest or restraint of an excitatory process.

Keypoints Parts of the body, manual direction of which will elicit or facilitate normal automatic movement responses.

L The left-hand side of the body.

Limbic system A term loosely applied to a group of brain structures associated with autonomic functions and certain aspects of emotion and behaviour.

μs Microsecond, one-millionth of a second.

Maturation Maturing of the system.

Modality Method of application, or employment, of a therapeutic agent.

Monosynaptic Nerve pathway having only one synapse.

Morbidity Incidence or prevalence of a disease.

Morphological Pertaining to the form and structure of a particular organism.

Motility Ability to move freely without external aid.

MRI Magnetic Resonance Imaging.

MUAP Motor Unit Action Potential, the natural electrical frequency at which a muscle motor unit normally receives action potentials from its motoneuron pool.

N The non-stroke, unaffected, side of the body.

Neuromuscular plasticity The responsive nature of the neuromuscular systems – including the central nervous system – to physiological stressing.

Neuron Nerve cell.

Neurotrophins Intraneural hormones.

Oedema Swelling caused by fluid in the tissues.

Orthosis Orthopaedic appliance or apparatus used to support, align, prevent or correct deformities or to improve the function of movable parts of the body.

Osteoporosis Loss of bone density.

Oxidative Richly oxygenated.

Paradigm A concept or theory generally held to be true.

Parametric specification Contextual and task-specific memory enabling functional activity, e.g. to gauge the force and direction of movement required for a successful action.

PAS A computerized Patient Administration System.

Perception Understanding, mental interpretation of a sensory stimulus.

Peripatetic Itinerant, travelling.

Peripheral Away from the centre, e.g. the limbs.

Peristalsis The travelling wave-like contractions in smooth muscle which propel food through the gut.

Perseveration Persistence or repetition of the same response after the causative stimulus has ceased, or in response to different stimuli.

Perturbation Disturbance to the stable base during movement.

Phasic A transient state, muscle fibres coded for fast response.

PET Positron Emission Tomography.

Phenotype Gene expression; the physical, biochemical and physiological coding determined genetically and environmentally.

Philogenetic Relationship based on closeness of evolutionary descent.

Phonological store A memory system utilizing an 'inner ear' for recognizing sound.

Physiological stressing Repetition of the same stimuli for long enough to produce changes in the neuromuscular systems.

Polysynaptic Having more than one synapse.

POMR Problem Orientated Medical Recording.

Pragmatism Doctrine which tests the truth of a concept by its results in practice.

Premorbid Before the development of the disease.

Procedural learning The acquisition of mental and physical skills.

Proprioception Sensation in the joints and tendons indicating position of the limb and direction of movement.

Protocols Rules of procedure.

PSR Positive Supporting Reflex, a push-off action from the ball of the foot incorporating the 'extensor thrust' position with ankle plantarflexion and inversion, knee extension, slight flexion at the hip and the up and backwards twist of the pelvis.

Pushers Strokes whose automatic equilibrium and supporting reactions are only initiated unilaterally – on the N side – so that they push themselves over to the S (hemiplegic) side when trying to maintain or recover their balance.

Quadrupod Adjustable-height walking stick ending in four legs.

R The right-hand side of the body.

Reciprocal innervation Interaction of muscles around a joint to enable fluency of movement – as the prime movers are stimulated to contract, the opposing group relaxes to the same degree at the same rate.

RIND Reversible Ischaemic Neurological Deficit, a stroke which lasts longer than 24 hours but recovers within 7 days, leaving no immediately obvious disability.

Rollator Walking frame with wheels on the front legs, for pushing – instead of lifting – forwards.

S The stroke-affected side of the body.

Sarcomere The contractile unit of myofibrils.

Semantic memory Acquired or learned 'general' knowledge.

Sensory extinction Failure to recognize stimuli on the S side when the same stimulus is presented simultaneously to the N side, although the stimulus can be recognized when presented to the S side only.

Serial ordering Planning of sequential movements for functional activity.

Shoulder-hand syndrome A flaccid arm and hand, sometimes painful, showing poor circulation and often accompanied by subluxation of the shoulder joint. The hand feels cold and damp and there can be hyperextension at the knuckles.

Somatic system The part of the nervous system that controls the striated muscle tissue for physical activity.

Spasticity Persistent increased muscle tone in the stereotyped reflex patterns, preventing normal movement.

Sphincter A ring-like band of muscle fibres that constricts a passage or closes a natural orifice.

STARS A structured functional assessment system now marketed as computer software.

Stereotyped reflex Persistent non-functional movement pattern.

Sub-cortical Below the cerebral cortex.

Sub-cortical approach Strategy to elicit automatic movement responses when selective movement is difficult to initiate.

Substratum Underlying basis.

Symmetrical tonic neck reflex Forward flexion of the head triggers flexion of both upper limbs with extension of both lower limbs.

Synapse The site of functional apposition between neurons and between neurons and effector organs, across which impulses are transmitted by electrical and/or chemical polarization.

Synergists The muscles around a joint which stabilize it to allow movement to take place at other joints, e.g. the shoulder is stabilized for hand dexterity.

Tactile Of, by or affecting the sense of touch, skin sensation.

Thalamic pain Hypersensitivity or pain affecting all or part of the S-side of the body. The thalamus is seldom the source of the problem, but the sympathetic tracts of the autonomic nervous system are always involved.

Thrombus Blood clot.

TIA Transient Ischaemic Attack, a stroke which lasts less than 24 hours with no lasting effects.

Tonic A maintained, sustained or static state, muscle fibres coded for strength, e.g. to support the body against gravity.

Trophic code Genetic protein code.

Two-point discrimination A test for equality of sensation at both points when the same stimulation is applied simultaneously to two points in the same area of skin.

Unilateral neglect Lack of awareness of activity in or to the S side.

US UltraSound.

VH Variable Height (beds, plinths, tables).

Viscera Internal organs of the body, e.g. abdominal contents.

Visuospatial The visual interpretation of space.

Visuospatial sketch pad A memory system used in creating and manipulating visual images.

Voiding Emptying the bladder.

Waiter's tip reflex The arm is pulled across the front of the body and rotated inwards, with elbow extended and wrist flexed.

Working memory An alliance of temporary ('immediate memory') storage systems coordinated by an attentional component (the 'central executive').

Recommended reading

Selected literature relevant to stroke and rehabilitation. Books written by Strokes, and those written specifically for non-medically-trained readers, are listed towards the end.

Ada, L. and Canning, C. (eds) (1990) *Key Issues in Neurological Physiotherapy*, Heinemann Medical, Oxford.

Atkinson, R.L., Atkinson, R.C., Smith, E.E. and Bem, D.J. (1990) *Introduction to Psychology*, 10th edn, Harcourt Brace Jovanovich, Florida. Includes the biological basis of psychology, the organization of the nervous system – and lovely illustrations.

Bach-y-Rita, P. (Ed.) (1980) *Recovery of Function*, Hans Huber, Bern.

Barr, M.L. and Keenan, J.A. (1979) *Human Nervous System*, 5th edn, Harper International, New York.

Bobath, B. (1971) *Abnormal Postural Reflex Activity caused by Brain Lesions*, Heinemann, London.

Bobath, B. (1990) *Adult Hemiplegia*, 3rd edn, Heinemann, London.

Carr, J.H. and Shepherd, R.B. (1987) *A Motor Relearning Programme for Stroke*, 2nd edn, Heinemann Medical, Oxford.

Davies, P.M. (1985) *Steps to Follow – A Guide to the Treatment of Adult Hemiplegia*, Springer-Verlag, Berlin.

Davies, P.M. (1990) *Right in the Middle – Selective Trunk Activity*, Springer-Verlag, Berlin.

Eccles, J.C. (1980) *The Understanding of the Brain*, McGraw–Hill Book Company, London.

Eggers, O. (1983) *Occupational Therapy in the Treatment of Adult Hemiplegia*, William Heinemann Medical Books, London.

Ellis, A.W. and Young, A.W. (1988) *Human Cognitive Neuropsychology*, Lawrence Erlbaum Associates, Hove.

Garoutte, B. (1987) *Survey of Functional Neuroanatomy*, 2nd edn, Jones Medical Publications, Greenbrae, California.

Goodglass, H. and Kaplan, E. (1976) *The Assessment of Aphasia and Related Disorders*, Lea & Febiger, Boston.

Gordon, W.A. (ed.) (1993) *Advances in Stroke Rehabilitation*, Andover Medical Publications, Boston. With the exception of several outdated comments on rehabilitation and recovery in the first two chapters!

Hart, N. (1985) *The Sociology of Health and Medicine*, Causeway books, Ormskirk.

Humphreys, G.W. and Riddoch, M.J. (1987) *To See But Not To See – A Case Study of Visual Agnosia*, Lawrence Erlbaum Associates, London.

Kapit, W. and Elson, L.M. (1977) *The Anatomy Coloring Book*, Harper Collins, New York. A delightful learning experience!

Kidd, G., Lawes, N. and Musa, I. (1992) *Understanding Neuromuscular Plasticity*, Edward Arnold, Sevenoaks.

Logemann, J. (1983) *Evaluation and Treatment of Swallowing Disorders*, College Hill Press, California.

Miller, N. (1986) *Dyspraxia and its Management*, Croom Helm, London.

Palastanga, N., Field, D. and Soames, R. (1989) *Anatomy and Movement*, Butterworth–Heinemann, London.

Ross, K. and Wilson, K.J.W. (1990) *Anatomy and Physiology in Health and Illness*, 7th edn, Churchhill Livingstone, London.

Skelly, M. (1979) *Amer-Ind Gestural Code*, Elsevier Science, Barking.

Stein, J.F. (1987) *An Introduction to Neurophysiology*, Blackwell Scientific Publications, Oxford.

Thompson, S.B.N. and Morgan, M. (1989) *Occupational Therapy for Stroke Rehabilitation*, Chapman & Hall, London.

Wertz, R., La Pointe, L. and Rosenbek, J. (1984) *Apraxia of Speech in Adults*, Grune & Stratton, London.

Wilson, B. and Moffat, N. (eds) (1984) *Clinical Management of Memory Problems*, Croom Helm, London.

Wood, R.Ll. and Fussey, I. (eds) (1990) *Cognitive Rehabilitation in Perspective*, Taylor & Francis, London.

GENERAL READING

Edelman, G. and Greenwood, R. (eds) (1992) *Jumbly Words, and Rights Where Wrongs Should Be: The experience of aphasia from the inside*, Far Communications, Kibworth.

Lynch, M. and Grisogono, V. (1991) *Strokes and Head Injuries – A Guide for Patients, Families, Friends and Carers*, John Murray, London.

Sarton, M. (1988) *After the Stroke – a journal*, The Women's Press, London.

Swaffield, L. (1990) *Stroke – The Complete Guide to Recovery and Rehabilitation*, Thorsons, Wellingborough.

Youngson, R.M. (1987) *Stroke! A Self-help Manual for Stroke Sufferers and Their Relatives*, David & Charles, Newton Abbot.

Reading is to the mind what exercise is to the body.

(Sir Richard Steele)

Index

Page numbers appearing in **bold** refer to figures.